# Study and Review for

# *E M T*

# *PREHOSPITAL*

# *CARE*

# Study and Review for

# E M T

## PREHOSPITAL

## CARE

## Mark C. Henry, MD

Associate Professor and Chairman
Department of Emergency Medicine
School of Medicine
State University of New York at Stony Brook
Stony Brook, New York

## Edward R. Stapleton, EMT-P

Director of Prehospital Care and Education
University Hospital
Instructor
Department of Emergency Medicine
School of Medicine
State University of New York at Stony Brook
Stony Brook, New York

**W.B. SAUNDERS COMPANY**
Harcourt Brace Jovanovich, Inc.

W.B. Saunders Company
Harcourt Brace Jovanovich, Inc.
The Curtis Center
Independence Square West
Philadelphia, PA 19106

*Editor:* Margaret M. Biblis
*Developmental Editor:* Shirley Kuhn
*Designer:* Paul Fry
*Production Manager:* Carolyn Naylor
*Illustration Specialist:* Cecelia Roberts

Study and Review for EMT: Prehospital Care                                     0-7216-4618-2

Copyright © 1992 by W.B. Saunders Company

Printed in United States of America

Last digit is the print number: 9   8   7   6   5   4   3   2

# Study and Review Guide for EMT: Prehospital Care

The Study and Review Guide for EMT: Prehospital Care is designed to provide the reader of the related textbook with the opportunity to reinforce and evaluate the knowledge and skills learned in the classroom and during reading. It also is useful for any EMT student or refresher candidate preparing for program and certifying exams.

The guide includes both multiple choice and matching questions that evaluate and reinforce basic information or the so-called enabling objectives of learning. Multiple choice and matching items were utilized to simulate the most common formats used in program and certifying examinations. These items are designed to provide the essential knowledge needed to understand and remember key building blocks of information that lay the foundation for clinical application.

Multiple choice and matching questions are followed by case histories that provide an opportunity to practice clinical application, synthesis (providing information in new ways) and analysis (performing evaluations and assessments) of critical situations. Case histories provide you the opportunity to practice the critical thinking needed to make assessment, treatment and transport decisions in prehospital care. You should first read the case history and imagine yourself at the scene. Make the assessment and decide on a treatment and transport plan, then review questions. By using this approach you will begin to prepare yourself for clinical performance.

Finally there are skills performance sheets for the essential skills learned in class and during your reading. These skill sheets are adapted from state and national agencies and reflect the state-of-the-art performance standards. However, you should check with your program instructor to see if there are customized program skill sheets before using the approach in the study and review guide. A practical method for reinforcing skills is to make a brief list of the procedure steps prior to reviewing the skills performance sheets. Then compare your list to the study guide sheet for confirmation or clarification. If the skill requires minimal equipment and is safe to practice at home (i.e., patient assessment), have a family member, friend or classmate observe and check off your performance. This is a valuable way to maximize your classroom time.

How to Use This Book

There are several learning strategies that can be adopted depending on your background. For example, if you are a refresher candidate and have worked in prehospital care for several years, you can take each chapter exam, score the exam with the answer key in the back of the book and review material as needed.

If you are a new student, you may want to use the following approach to ensure an efficient and effective learning process:

1.   Read the chapter carefully as prescribed in the preface of EMT: Prehospital Care; review the chapter objectives, skim the chapter and main headings, read the review questions at the end of the chapter and

take the chapter exam.  Use the answer sheet to check your understanding of the material.

2.      After taking the exam, score it using the answer key in the back of the book and review the necessary material.

3.      Read the case histories. Again, picture yourself at the scene while reading the case and prior to answering the questions.  Use the information in the case history to make the appropriate assessment and treatments, then answer the related questions.

4.      At the end of each chapter, review the skill performance sheets in the manner described above.

Since your EMT program may be given over a long period of time (up to several months) you should retake the exams at standard intervals.  Toward the end of the program, conduct one final review of the entire study guide.  When you take the final practice test, **budget approximately 1 minute per question**.  This will help you to develop a pace suitable for the final program examination and the state certifying examination.

As a rule you should skip over questions for which the answers are unclear and return to them at the end of a chapter.  Failure to follow this process will cost you valuable time and increase your adrenaline level during the testing process. Obviously, it is important to return to the items at the end of a test to ensure that no question is overlooked.  A final review of the answer sheet should be a routine practice for any test taker.

Don't be discouraged if you don't score high on your first try.  We have intentionally included some higher level questions to build up your "academic strength" for the final exam.  By being familiar with concepts at a level of understanding, you will feel confident when faced with the typical basic level question on a state certifying exam.

Remember, true learning is a **long-lasting change in behavior** and retention of information depends on:

1.      Understanding the concepts related to the material
2.      Periodic reinforcement
3.      A constant dedication to continuing education

We hope that you find this study and review guide and the related textbook interesting and relevant during your educational endeavors, and we wish you success and many rewarding EMS experiences.

We wish to thank Eric Niegelberg for his invaluable assistance in the development of test items for this work and the related Instructor's Guide.  A special thank you to the Laerdal Medical Corporation for use of the ECG strips contained within chapter six.

Mark C. Henry, MD
Edward R. Stapleton, EMT-P

# CONTENTS

*Chapter 1*

## INTRODUCTION TO PREHOSPITAL EMERGENCY CARE

1. A system of resources and personnel necessary to provide immediate care to the ill and injured describes a(n):

   a. emergency medical service system
   b. ambulance service
   c. enhanced 911 dispatching system
   d. hospital emergency service

2. Much of the growth and technical development of prehospital emergency care can be attributed to methods developed:

   a. during disaster drills
   b. by outpatient clinics
   c. during war
   d. during laboratory animal research

3. The Civil War is noted for the first use in the United States of:

   a. MAST trousers
   b. MASH units
   c. ambulances
   d. a formal system of triage

4. The Korean War saw the first use of:

   a. large bore IVs to stabilize the patient in the field
   b. large hospital ships to provide definitive care to all patients
   c. physicians assigned to every platoon
   d. helicopters to provide rapid transport of casualties

5. Michael Reese Hospital in Chicago is credited with the first use of:

   a. horse drawn ambulances
   b. motorized ambulances
   c. MAST trousers
   d. emergency medical technicians (EMT's)

6. The leading cause of trauma deaths is attributed to:

   a. electrocution
   b. automobile accidents
   c. falls
   d. burn injuries

1

7.   In 1966 a landmark paper entitled "Accidental Death and Disability: The Neglected Diseases of Modern Society" was published by the:

a. Department of Transportation (DOT)
b. American Medical Association
c. National Academy of Sciences
d. U.S. Surgeon General

8.   The leading cause of death in the United States is:

a. cancer
b. diabetes
c. heart disease
d. trauma

9.   Approximately 350,000 deaths occur outside the hospital each year in the U.S. due to:

a. myocardial infarction
b. electrocution
c. burn injuries
d. AIDS

10.   Lay rescuers, first responders, EMTs and paramedics, emergency departments, intensive care units, etc., are all components of a(n):

a. EMS system
b. health care agency
c. emergency network
d. crisis intervention team

11.   All of the following are primary responsibilities of an EMT at the scene of an accident except:

a. emergency care
b. patient assessment
c. disentanglement
d. immobilization

12.   The hospital's emergency department, which is a component of an EMS system, is the "intersection of care" for the critical patient because it:

a. provides definitive care to a patient prior to discharge
b. trains the public in CPR and first aid
c. provides stabilizing measures prior to transfer to the operating room or critical care unit
d. coordinates multiple components of every EMS system

13.   The lay rescuer is someone who:

    a.     is not a part of the EMS system
    b.     can never provide CPR and first aid for the patient
    c.     treats the patient in the emergency department
    d.     is often the first help the patient has

14.   Categorization, a method of hospital designation, is determined according to the:

    a.     location of the hospital
    b.     capabilities in different areas of care
    c.     preferences of the public
    d.     size of the hospital

15.   The EMS act of 1973 provided funding for the development of EMS systems throughout the country. This legislation defined all of the following except _____ as components of an EMS system.

    a.     training
    b.     communications
    c.     accessibility of care
    d.     alteration of care

16.   This stage of an EMS system provides long-term care designed to restore the function of the body.

    a.     rehabilitation units
    b.     emergency departments
    c.     operating room
    d.     outpatient units

17.   This stage of an EMS system provides definitive care and is cited as the end point of the "golden hour." There are various types of these units to account for different types of critically ill or injured patients.

    a.     rehabilitation units
    b.     emergency departments
    c.     operating room
    d.     outpatient units

18.   This component of an EMS system coordinates resources and allows EMS providers to communicate with one another. It allows for on-line medical control and brings specialized help to the scene an accident or illness.

    a.     headquarters
    b.     ambulance
    c.     command center
    d.     communications system

19.     The dispatch system is the:

    a.      component of the system that receives the call for help, sends the appropriate vehicles and coordinates resources
    b.      physician staffed control center to advise on patient treatment
    c.      transmission of EKG data from the patient in the field to the physician at the base hospital
    d.      portable radios that are carried to the scene of an emergency

Match the EMS system role in column B to the description in column A

| Column A | | Column B | |
|---|---|---|---|
| **B** 20. | the intersection of care | a. | first responder |
| **F** 21. | usually the first medical person to see the patient | b. | emergency department |
| **A** 22. | provides initial care (i.e., CPR) with minimal equipment | c. | critical care unit |
| | | d. | rehabilitation |
| *d* 23. | returns patient to function within the community | e. | communications |
| | | f. | EMT |
| *e* 24. | notification, prioritizing, calls, dispatch, etc., occur through this system | | |

25.     Biotelemetry is:

    a.      continuous EKG monitor worn by some cardiac patients
    b.      utilization of satellite transceivers to dispatch cardiac data to hospitals
    c.      implantable device used by some cardiac patients to properly pace the heart
    d.      transmission of EKG data from the patient in the field to the physician at the base hospital

26.     Physician involvement and participation in all phases of the EMS system to ensure quality care best defines the concept of:

    a.      categorization
    b.      standardization
    c.      systemization
    d.      medical control

27. Medical control of prehospital care should include:

    a. needs assessment of the system
    b. training and certification
    c. protocol development
    d. all of the above

28. Patient assessment, patient care and transfer of the patient to hospital staff are:

    a. beyond the scope of practice of the EMT
    b. primary roles of the EMT in most systems
    c. acts that must be completed and documented to prevent an act of negligence
    d. taken together form the basis for malfeasance

Indicate which of the roles of the EMT listed in column A are primary versus secondary (other) in most systems. Column B items can be used more than once.

| Column A | Column B |
| --- | --- |
| 29. patient assessment | a. primary |
| 30. extrication | b. secondary (other) |
| 31. patient care | |
| 32. transfer of the patient to hospital staff | |

33. A serious effort to acquire the requisite skills taught in the initial EMT training program, as well as a continued effort to prevent deterioration of knowledge is the best way to maintain:

    a. respect
    b. competence
    c. certification
    d. analytical skills

34. "Acting requisite to the body of knowledge which defines the service and abilities of the professional...according to the oath of the profession. Historical first to religious vows...." This definition best describes the term:

    a. competence
    b. professionalism
    c. ethics
    d. honorable

5

35. The person who may provide electrical therapy (and no other advanced skills) to a patient in cardiac arrest best describes:

    a. EMT-Paramedic
    c. EMT-Ambulance
    c. EMT-Defibrillation
    d. EMT-Intermediate

36. The person who usually is the first medical person to see the patient best describes the:

    a. physician
    b. EMT
    c. lay rescuer
    d. nurse

37. The person who interprets the EKG, performs invasive airway skills and has a more broadly based knowledge of pharmacology best describes the:

    a. EMT-Paramedic
    b. EMT-Ambulance
    c. EMT-Defibrillation
    d. EMT-Intermediate

38. The person who provides advanced airway management, IV therapy and possibly limited drug administration best describes the:

    a. EMT-Paramedic
    b. EMT-Ambulance
    c. EMT-Defibrillation
    d. EMT-Intermediate

39. You have completed the treatment and transportation of a patient who sustained a gunshot wound to the chest. Upon leaving the hospital you are approached by a reporter from the local newspaper. You may tell the reporter:

    a. the vital signs of the patient
    b. that the patient is all right and give the
       reporter a copy of the ambulance call report
    c. only that the patient was shot and that he is in
       the hospital
    d. the past medical history as told to you by the
       patient

40. The body of knowledge, laws, policies, standards and guidelines set forth by various standard-setting organizations that provides the basis of prehospital care, along with the everyday practice of other providers, best describes:

    a. values of practice
    b. the standard of care
    c. emergency laws
    d. competence

41. Standard of Care is defined by which of the following?

    a. DOT curriculum
    b. local medical protocols
    c. textbooks of prehospital care
    d. all of the above

42. A duty to act, a breach of duty, an injury to the patient and a causal connection between the injury and the EMT's actions are all ingredients of:

    a. abandonment
    b. a malpractice case
    c. malfeasance
    d. an EMS system

43. In many states, the medical practice act addresses all of the following except:

    a. scope of practice for emergency medical services personnel
    b. minimum training standards for personnel
    c. medical control issues
    d. trauma center designation

44. Your ambulance is on the scene of a 72 year old female who tripped on the curb and injured her hip. You inform her of the benefits and consequences of the care provided. She is being treated under the concept of _____ consent.

    a. implied
    b. applied
    c. informed
    d. presumed

45. Your ambulance is on the scene of a 54 year old female patient who is having a heart attack. During treatment of this patient you hear another call for a child who is choking approximately one mile away. If you leave your patient and respond to the child who is choking you may be guilty of:

    a. malfeasance
    b. abandonment
    c. negligence
    d. breach of duty

7

46. Your ambulance is dispatched to the scene of a "man down." Upon arrival you find a 52 year old unconscious patient. Treatment may be rendered under the concept of _____ consent.

    a. informed
    b. presumed
    c. implied
    d. surrogate

47. An emancipated minor is a(n):

    a. individual who is under the legal adult age but who is living independently of the parent
    b. child who is injured at school and the parent is at work
    c. patient who has been judged mentally incompetent by the court
    d. individual who is under the legal adult age but who is injured while working

48. Good Samaritan laws are designed to protect the:

    a. EMT against legal action due to abandonment of the patient
    b. EMT against legal action due to gross negligence in the driving of the ambulance
    c. EMT against legal action if CPR is not started on a patient in witnessed cardiac arrest and who is pronounced dead at the scene
    d. private citizen who is functioning in a nonprofessional capacity and without an expectation of remuneration

49. Rigor mortis, decapitation and extreme dependent lividity are acceptable criteria for:

    a. rapid transport to the hospital
    b. requesting a physician to the scene to assist in patient care
    c. withholding CPR
    d. bypassing the local community hospital and transporting the patient to the nearest trauma center

50. Which of the following is acceptable criteria for withholding CPR?

    a. 15 minute history of cardiac arrest
    b. 20 minute history of cardiac arrest
    c. 30 minute history of cardiac arrest
    d. extreme dependent lividity

## Chapter 2

## ANATOMY, PHYSIOLOGY AND PATIENT ASSESSMENT

Match the definition in column B to the correct term in column A.

| Column A | | Column B | |
|---|---|---|---|
| b 1. | medial | a. | toward the rear of the body |
| e 2. | proximal | b. | toward midline |
| f 3. | superior | c. | lying facedown |
| a 4. | posterior | d. | movement away from the body |
| c 5. | prone | e. | toward the point of origin |
| d 6. | abduction | f. | toward the head |

7.     The study of structure or form of living things is called:

    a.    anatomy
    b.    physics
    c.    biology
    d.    physiology

8.     Which of the following is a function of the skeletal system?

    a.    gives structure and support
    b.    produces plasma
    c.    destroys red blood cells
    d.    initiates respiration

9.     In the normal anatomical position, the body is erect with feet together and parallel, arms extended, and palms and head facing:

    a.    medially
    b.    posteriorly
    c.    anteriorly
    d.    laterally

10.     The heart, great vessels, esophagus and trachea are located in which of the following body spaces?

    a.    pleura
    b.    peritoneal cavity
    c.    mediastinum
    d.    pelvic cavity

Match the type of spinal vertebrae in column A to the correct number found in the human spine in column B.

| Column A | | Column B | |
|---|---|---|---|
| c 11. | cervical vertebrae | a. | 12 mobile |
| a 12. | thoracic vertebrae | b. | 5 fused |
| e 13. | lumbar vertebrae | c. | 7 mobile |
| b 14. | sacral | d. | 4 fused |
| d 15. | coccyx | e. | 5 mobile |

16. The ilium, ischium and pubis collectively form the:

    a. shoulder girdle
    b. pelvic girdle
    c. thoracic cage
    d. metacarpal bones

17. The abdominal quadrants are created by two intersecting lines that meet at the:

    a. xiphoid process
    b. epigastric region
    c. umbilicus
    d. pubic bone

Match the function in column B to the type of muscle in column A.

| Column A | | Column B | |
|---|---|---|---|
| a 18. | voluntary or skeletal muscle | a. | movement of arms |
| c 19. | involuntary or smooth muscle | b. | pumping of blood |
| b 20. | cardiac muscle | c. | digestion |

21. The respiratory structure responsible for preventing aspiration of food and other materials into the airway is called the:

    a. bronchiole
    b. carina
    c. pharynx
    d. epiglottis

22. The movement of oxygen from the lungs to the blood occurs at the level of the:

    a. bronchi
    b. alveoli
    c. trachea
    d. larynx

23. The pumping chambers of the heart that deliver blood to the lungs and body tissues are called the:

    a. septums
    b. sinuses
    c. atria
    d. ventricles

24. The major artery that delivers blood to the body or systemic circulation is called the:

    a. aorta
    b. pulmonary
    c. coronary
    d. vena cava

25. The type of vessel that permits diffusion to take place, and that is one cell thick is called a:

    a. capillary
    b. vein
    c. arteriole
    d. artery

26. The type of blood cell that is responsible for combating infection is called:

    a. red blood cell
    b. white blood cell
    c. platelet
    d. plasma

27. The protein that is responsible for the transport of oxygen and carbon dioxide is called:

    a. plasma
    b. thrombin
    c. hemoglobin
    d. fibrinogen

28. Which of the following is part of the central nervous system?

    a. spinal cord
    b. brain
    c. peripheral nerves
    d. both a and b

29. The part of the brain responsible for balance and coordination is called the:

    a. cerebrum
    b. pons
    c. medulla
    d. cerebellum

30. The body system concerned with maintaining homeostasis, influencing growth, reproduction and response to stress through the release of hormones is called the:

    a. digestive system
    b. circulatory system
    c. endocrine system
    d. lymphatic system

31. The organ responsible for the release of insulin, which allows for the metabolism of glucose, is the :

    a. liver
    b. gallbladder
    c. pancreas
    d. spleen

32. The largest part of the digestive tract, where absorption of nutrients occurs, is called the:

    a. esophagus
    b. liver
    c. small intestine
    d. rectum

33. The urinary system tube responsible for transporting urine from the bladder to the external opening of both the male and female genitalia is called the:

    a. ureter
    b. urethra
    c. common bile duct
    d. prostate

34.     The tube that connects the ovary to the uterus is called the:

    a.     fallopian tube
    b.     cervix
    c.     ovarian tubule
    d.     uterine duct

35.     The heart, lung and brain are dependent upon one another to maintain vital functions. Which of the following reasons best explains why a patient stops breathing following a cardiac arrest?

    a.     hypoxia to the brain stem
    b.     loss of voluntary breathing control
    c.     damage to the cerebrum
    b.     toxicity of blood

36.     Clinical death is defined as:

    a.     no pulse and no respirations
    b.     brain death
    c.     biological death of the heart
    d.     unexpected death

Match the phase of patient assessment in column B to the appropriate component in column A. Column B items can be used more than once.

| Column A | | Column B | |
|---|---|---|---|
| 37. | extremity examination | a. | dispatch review |
| 38. | carotid pulse check | b. | scene survey |
| 39. | head tilt-chin lift | c. | primary survey |
| 40. | mechanism of injury | d. | secondary survey |
| 41. | plan route | | |
| 42. | past medical history | | |

43.     Gathering information from bystanders, identifying hazards, securing the scene and calling for specialized assistance are all components of the:

    a.     primary survey
    b.     scene survey
    c.     secondary survey
    d.     dispatch review

44.   After establishing unresponsiveness in a prone trauma patient you should:

a.   leave the patient in the prone position and continue with your survey
b.   logroll the patient to the lateral recumbent position and continue with your survey
c.   logroll the patient to the supine position and continue with your survey
d.   leave the patient in the prone position and transport immediately

45.   Tilting the head back with one hand while lifting the lower margin of the jaw with the index and middle fingers of the other hand best describes the:

a.   jaw thrust without head tilt
b.   chin pull maneuver
c.   head tilt-neck lift
d.   head tilt-chin lift

46.   The best method for evaluating the adequacy of ventilation is by:

a.   observing chest rise
b.   placing a mirror near the mouth and nose
c.   feeling the chest wall for expansion
d.   checking the pulse rate

47.   Cyanosis, accessory muscle use and deviated trachea are all signs noted in the _____ assessment within the primary survey.

a.   circulatory
b.   neurological
c.   respiratory
d.   secondary

48.   The correct location of palpation for the carotid pulse is:

a.   at groove between the larynx and muscle in the neck
b.   at the angle of the jaw adjacent to the muscle
c.   just above the suprasternal notch
d.   just above the clavicle, adjacent to the trachea

49.   The American Heart Association recommends that the carotid pulse be palpated on:

a.   either side of the neck
b.   the side opposite the rescuer
c.   the same side as the rescuer
d.   both sides of the neck each time

50. The American Heart Association recommends that the carotid pulse be palpated <u>initially</u> for:

   a. 2-3 seconds
   b. 5-7 seconds
   c. 5-10 seconds
   d. 10-20 seconds

51. Capillary refill is considered delayed when refill takes more than:

   a. 0.5 seconds
   b. 1.0 seconds
   c. 1.5 seconds
   d. 2.0 seconds

Match the pulse point in column A to the approximate minimum blood pressure (when the pulse is still palpable) in column B.

| Column A | Column B |
| --- | --- |
| 52. carotid | a. 60 systolic |
| 53. radial | b. 70 systolic |
| 54. femoral | c. 80 systolic |

55. The "V" of the AVPU evaluation of mental state refers to a patient's ability to respond to:

   a. vigorous stimuli
   b. verbal stimuli
   c. visual stimuli
   d. vivid stimuli

56. Which of the following questions reflects the best way to inquire about a chest pain complaint in a medical history?

   a. Was your chest pain squeezing in nature?
   b. How would you describe the pain in your own words?
   c. Did it feel like someone was standing on your chest?
   d. Was the pain viselike in nature?

57. The expression of the patient's main complaint in his or her own words is called the:

   a. history of present illness
   b. primary problem
   c. primary complaint
   d. chief complaint

58. The sequence of events, activity at the onset of the problem, location and radiation of pain, and aggravating and relieving factors are examples of the:

    a. history of present illness
    b. past medical history
    c. primary survey
    d. chief complaint

59. The four major diseases (the big four) that are routinely inquired about during the past medical history with older adult patients are:

    a. heart disease, epilepsy, chronic obstructive pulmonary disease, high blood pressure
    b. heart disease, diabetes, cancer, high blood pressure
    c. diabetes, chronic obstructive pulmonary disease, high blood pressure, stroke
    d. heart disease, diabetes, chronic obstructive pulmonary disease, high blood pressure

60. The normal range of respiratory rate in the adult is approximately _____ per minute.

    a. 5-15
    b. 10-15
    c. 12-20
    d. 15-25

Match the respiratory sound in column A with the likely underlying problem in column B.

| Column A | | Column B |
| --- | --- | --- |
| 61. gurgling | a. | obstruction by the tongue |
| 62. snoring | b. | fluid in the airway |
| 63. wheezing | c. | narrowed lower airway |
| 64. stridor | d. | narrowed upper airway |

65. The artery routinely utilized to monitor the rate, regularity and quality of the pulse is the:

    a. radial
    b. femoral
    c. brachial
    d. ulna

66. The normal range of pulse rate for an adult at rest is approximately _____ per minute.

    a. 40-60
    b. 50-70
    c. 60-80
    d. 80-100

67. The blood pressure is determined by the resistance provided by the blood vessels (peripheral vascular resistance) times the:

    a. pulse rate
    b. pulse pressure
    c. stroke
    d. cardiac output

68. Blood pressure determined by listening through a stethoscope is called blood pressure by:

    a. auscultation
    b. palpation
    c. oscillation
    d. vibration

69. The artery that is routinely monitored while listening for a blood pressure is the _____ artery.

    a. radial
    b. brachial
    c. ulna
    d. femoral

70. The first sound heard when listening for a blood pressure that reflects the contraction phase of the heart is called the _____ pressure.

    a. diastolic
    d. systolic
    c. pulse
    d. contractile

71. A disadvantage of a blood pressure taken by palpation is that you can obtain only the _____ pressure.

    a. diastolic
    d. systolic
    c. pulse
    d. contractile

72.    The maximum score obtainable in the Glasgow coma scale is:

    a.    5
    b.    6
    c.    10
    d.    15

73.    "Raccoon eyes" and "Battle's sign" are both indicators of:

    a.    a potential skull fracture
    b.    certain brain damage
    c.    a broken nose
    d.    a fracture to the orbit bones

74.    The muscles used to determine the presence of respiratory distress are called the:

    a.    deltoid muscles
    b.    pectoral muscles
    c.    diaphragm muscles
    d.    accessory muscles

75.    Air beneath the skin that is characterized by a crackling sensation during palpation of the neck and upper chest is called:

    a.    pneumodermas rales
    b.    dermatitis pneumonia
    c.    subcutaneous emphysema
    d.    crepitant rales

76.    The structure that can be palpated midline above the sternum is called the:

    a.    esophagus
    b.    pharynx
    c.    glottis
    d.    trachea

77.    If you encounter an open wound of the chest wall during your assessment you should cover it with a(n):

    a.    multitrauma dressing
    b.    airtight dressing
    c.    4x4 dressing
    d.    pressure dressing

78.    Movement of a section of the chest wall in the opposite direction of the
       remaining chest wall during ventilation is called:

       a.    paradoxical breathing
       b.    thoracic deviation
       c.    mediastinal shift
       d.    thoracic paradoxis

79.    When palpating a painful abdomen you should begin:

       a.    at the site of pain
       b.    away from the site of pain
       c.    just lateral to the site
       d.    just medial to the site

80.    The iliac crests of the pelvis are palpated by gentle compression posteriorly
       and:

       a.    anteriorly
       b.    medially
       c.    laterally
       d.    superiorly

81.    The pelvis is also palpated at the:

       a.    sacrum
       b.    pubic symphysis
       c.    umbilicus
       d.    inguinal area

82.    When examining the lower extremities, you should compare:

       a.    one to the other
       b.    upper thighs to lower leg
       c.    them to the upper extremities
       d.    anterior-posterior diameter to the lateral

83.    The femoral pulse is located halfway between the anterior superior iliac spine
       and the:

       a.    umbilicus
       b.    sacrum
       c.    pubic symphysis
       d.    ischium

84.    The posterior tibial pulse is located behind the:

       a.    inner ankle bone (medial malleolus)
       b.    mid-thigh region
       c.    hip region
       d.    knee cap

85.    The bone that can be palpated on the anterior surface of the lower leg is the:

    a.    humerus
    b.    tibia
    c.    fibula
    d.    femur

86.    The pulse that can be palpated in the anterolateral aspect of the wrist just below the thumb is the:

    a.    brachial
    b.    ulna
    c.    radial
    d.    humeral

87.    Which of the following problems is most likely to result in an absent pulse in one arm:

    a.    a shock state with decreased perfusion
    b.    an obstruction of an artery by a bone end
    c.    hypotension due to arterial vasodilation
    d.    failure of the left side of the heart

88.    Having the patient flex and extend the foot, lift the leg and wiggle the toes most directly evaluates:

    a.    sensory function
    b.    mental state
    c.    motor function
    d.    brainstem function

89.    A patient with paralysis of the lower but not the upper extremities has most like injured the:

    a.    cervical spine
    b.    cerebrum
    c.    lumbar spine
    d.    brainstem

90.    Flexing the neck of a medical patient and finding stiffness is suggestive of irritation to the:

    a.    meninges (brain coverings)
    b.    brainstem
    c.    cerebrum
    d.    spinal cord

Skill Performance Sheet

# Patient Assessment

Student Name_____     Date_____

| Performance Standard | Performed | Failed |
|---|---|---|
| **PRIMARY SURVEY** | | |
| One EMT maintains in-line immobilization (if trauma patient) | | |
| Checks responsiveness | | |
| Opens airway with appropriate maneuver (head tilt-chin lift or jaw thrust) | | |
| Corrects problems with airway (i.e., suction) | | |
| Checks adequacy of breathing | | |
| Corrects problems with breathing (i.e., seals open chest wounds) | | |
| Checks pulse and adequacy of circulation | | |
| Corrects problems with circulation (i.e., bleeding control) | | |
| Evaluates disability (AVPU, pupils, motor and sensory) | | |
| Exposes patient (removes clothing) | | |
| **SECONDARY SURVEY** | | |
| Checks radial pulse | | |
| Takes blood pressure | | |
| Checks respiratory rate | | |
| Checks skin color and moisture | | |

CONTINUED ON NEXT PAGE

Skill Performance Sheet

## Patient Assessment (continued)

| Performance Standard | Performed | Failed |
|---|---|---|
| **HISTORY** | | |
| Chief complaint | | |
| History of present illness | | |
| Past medical history | | |
| Medications | | |
| Allergies | | |
| **HEAD TO TOE SURVEY** (Observes, Palpates, Listens) | | |
| Head (scalp, face, pupils, ears, nose mouth, Battle's sign) | | |
| Neck (vertebrae, trachea, neck veins, soft tissues) | | |
| Chest (anterior, lateral, posterior) | | |
| Breath sounds | | |
| Abdomen (anterior, lateral, posterior) | | |
| Pelvis (medial, posterior iliac crest and pubic symphysis palpation) | | |
| Buttocks | | |
| Extremities | | |

Comments_____

_____

_____

_____

Instructor _____     Circle One:  Pass  Fail

## Chapter 3

## RESPIRATORY EMERGENCIES

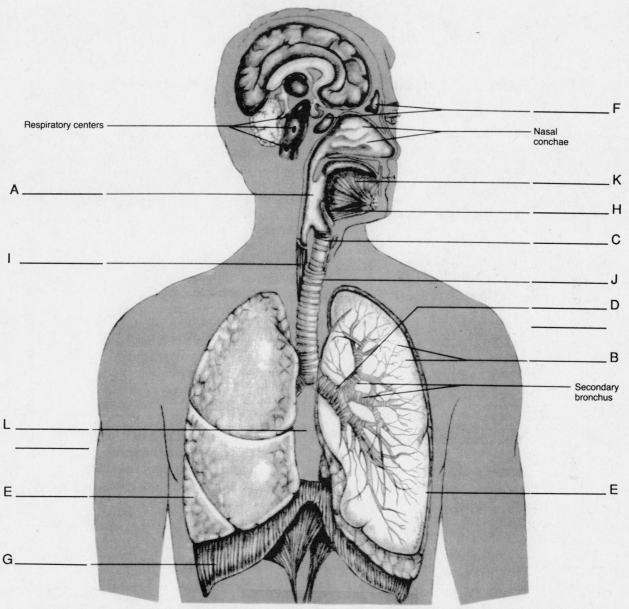

Respiratory centers

Nasal conchae

F

A

K

H

C

I

J

D

B

Secondary bronchus

L

E

E

G

(Solomon EP, Phillips GA: Understanding Human Anatomy and Physiology. Philadelphia, WB Saunders, 1987, p262)

Match the structures on the drawing above to the terms below:

A 1.  pharynx
L 2.  mediastinum
D 3.  primary bronchus
J 4.  trachea
B 5.  bronchioles
G 6.  diaphragm

C 7.  larynx
F 8.  sinuses
I 9.  esophagus
H 10. epiglottis
E 11. lung
K 12. tongue

13.    The structure that covers the trachea during swallowing to prevent aspiration is called the:

    a.     pharynx
    b.     epiglottis
    c.     thyroid cartilage
    d.     cricoid cartilage

14.    The respiratory structure that is palpable just above the sternum is the:

    a.     bronchus
    b.     trachea
    c.     carina
    d.     bronchiole

15.    The muscle that separates the chest and abdomen is called the:

    a.     diaphragm
    b.     intercostal
    c.     abdominis recti
    d.     none of the above

16.    The normal resting tidal volume for an adult is approximately:

    a.     500 ml
    b.     800 ml
    c.     1000 ml
    d.     2000 ml

17.    The process by which gases move from an area of higher concentration to an area of lower concentration is called:

    a.     ventilation
    b.     respiration
    c.     diffusion
    d.     transportation

18.    The portion of the lung where diffusion takes place is called the:

    a.     bronchi
    b.     pleura
    c.     bronchiole
    d.     alveoli

19. When the brainstem sends messages to the intercostals and diaphragm, they contract and increase the size of thoracic cavity. At that point, the pressure within the thoracic cavity _____, causing air to rush in.

    a. increases
    b. decreases
    c. remains the same
    d. none of the above

20. The substance secreted within the alveoli that is responsible for maintaining patent alveoli is called:

    a. pleural fluid
    b. mucus
    c. cilia
    d. surfactant

21. The maximum amount of air that can be expired after the maximum inspiration is called the:

    a. tidal volume
    b. vital capacity
    c. expiratory reserve
    d. total lung capacity

22. The amount of air inhaled and exhaled during a given breath is called the _____ volume.

    a. residual
    b. expiratory reserve
    c. total
    d. tidal

23. Normal atmospheric air contains approximately _____ oxygen.

    a. 15%
    b. 21%
    c. 28%
    d. 50%

24. In a normal respiratory system, the stimulus to breathe is related <u>primarily</u> to levels of:

    a. carbon dioxide
    b. oxygen
    c. blood volume
    d. none of the above

25.     The portion of the brain responsible for regulation of breathing is called the:

    a.     cerebrum
    b.     cerebellum
    c.     hypothalamus
    d.     brainstem

26.     A term commonly used to describe a feeling of shortness of breath is:

    a.     hemoptysis
    b.     tachypnea
    c.     dyspnea
    d.     ischemia

27.     Chest pain that occurs or is made worse by movement of the chest wall and breathing is called _____ chest pain.

    a.     pleuritic
    b.     dyspneic
    c.     ischemic
    d.     orthopneic

28.     A bluish discoloration of the skin caused by oxygen poor hemoglobin is called:

    a.     mottling
    b.     ecchymosis
    c.     cyanosis
    d.     anoxic erythema

29.     The term commonly used to describe the coughing up of blood is:

    a.     hematemesis
    b.     hematuria
    c.     hemoptysis
    d.     hemasputum

30.     The accessory muscles of inspiration are noted primarily by observing the:

    a.     chest wall
    b.     neck
    c.     abdominal wall
    d.     back

Match the breath sounds in column B with their normal location of auscultation in column A. One choice is extra.

| Column A | | Column B | |
|---|---|---|---|
| *B* 31. | top of the sternum and between the scapulas | a. | vesicular |
| *A* 32. | on the anterior, lateral and posterior chest walls | b. | bronchial |
| *C* 33. | upper and middle sternum and to its left and right borders | c. | bronchovesicular |
| | | d. | tracheal |

34. A high-pitched sound that is emitted from a narrowed upper airway and that usually occurs on inspiration is called:

    a.     wheeze
    b.     stridor
    c.     rhonchi
    d.     crackles

35. A high-pitched sound that is emitted from the lower airway that usually occurs on expiration and may be caused by asthma or COPD is called:

    a.     wheeze
    b.     stridor
    c.     rhonchi
    d.     crackles

36. During positive pressure ventilation, effective tidal volume is evaluated primarily on the basis of:

    a.     chest excursion
    b.     skin color
    c.     pupil response
    d.     none of the above

37. The most common complication of excessive or forceful ventilation is:

    a.     pneumothorax
    b.     gastric distention
    c.     oxygen toxicity
    d.     air embolism

38.   Which of the following administration devices results in the highest oxygen delivery to the patient?

    a.    nasal cannula
    b.    Venturi mask
    c.    nonrebreather mask
    d.    simple face mask

39.   In attempting to deliver 24% oxygen to a COPD patient the device of choice is the:

    a.    nonrebreather mask
    b.    simple face mask
    c.    Venturi mask
    d.    demand valve

40.   The most common cause of airway obstruction is:

    a.    allergic reactions
    b.    food
    c.    the tongue
    d.    trauma to the airway

41.   In patients with suspected spinal trauma, the manual airway maneuver of choice is the:

    a.    jaw thrust without head tilt
    b.    head tilt-neck lift
    c.    head tilt-chin lift
    d.    tongue pull

42.   The minimum tidal volume needed to effectively ventilate (see chest rise) an adult respiratory arrest victim is _____ ml of air.

    a.    500
    b.    800
    c.    1200
    d.    2000

43.   The correct ventilation rate for a nonbreathing adult patient is one breath every _____ seconds.

    a.    3
    b.    4
    c.    5
    d.    6

44. In the absence of spinal injury, the airway maneuver of choice is the:

    a. jaw thrust without head tilt
    b. head tilt-neck lift
    c. head tilt-chin lift
    d. tongue pull

45. Upon inserting an oropharyngeal airway, the patient begins to gag and choke. You next action should be to:

    a. remove the airway
    b. use a smaller airway
    c. lubricate the airway
    d. tape the airway in place

46. To ensure proper sizing, an oropharyngeal airway is measured from the center of the patient's mouth to the:

    a. angle of the jaw
    b. top of the ear
    c. cheek bone
    d. trachea

47. The pocket mask used in conjunction with 10-12 liters of oxygen per minute can result in maximum oxygen concentrations of approximately ___ %.

    a. 16
    b. 21
    c. 30
    d. 50

48. The major complication of a bag-valve-mask resuscitator is:

    a. overventilation and pneumothorax
    b. low tidal volumes due to errors in technique
    c. rupture of the bag during exhalation
    d. valve failure due to clogging

49. A bag-valve-mask used with an oxygen reservoir is capable of achieving a maximum of approximately _____ % oxygen delivery to the patient's airway.

    a. 25-35
    b. 50-60
    c. 75-80
    d. 90-100

50.　An oxygen cylinder is _____ to avoid confusion with other gases.

　　　a.　blue
　　　b.　purple
　　　c.　red
　　　d.　green

51.　The tank pressure of a full oxygen cylinder is usually _____ lb. per square inch.

　　　a.　700
　　　b.　1000
　　　c.　2000
　　　d.　4000

52.　The system used to avoid misplacement of a regulator on portable oxygen cylinders is called the:

　　　a.　oxygen cylinder safety system
　　　b.　pin index safety system
　　　c.　gas delivery safety system
　　　d.　regulator safety system

53.　Which of the following oxygen cylinders is the most portable?

　　　a.　D cylinder
　　　b.　E cylinder
　　　c.　H cylinder
　　　d.　M cylinder

54.　Regulators are designed to provide a safe pressure to the delivery device of approximately _____ PSI.

　　　a.　10-20
　　　b.　20-30
　　　c.　40-70
　　　d.　100-120

55.　A flowmeter that uses a gravity-controlled ball to measure the liter flow rates to the delivery device is called a _____ flowmeter.

　　　a.　bourdon gauge
　　　b.　pressure compensated
　　　c.　constant flow selector
　　　d.　double staged

Match the delivery device in column B to the appropriate oxygen concentrations in column A. One choice is extra.

Column A | Column B
---|---

*b* 56.   90% at 10-12 liters

a.   nasal cannula

*A* 57.   24-40% at 2-6 liters

b.   nonrebreather mask

*F* 58.   50-60% at 8-12 liters

d.   partial rebreather mask

e.   simple face mask

59.   Which of the following delivery devices is considered high flow?

    a.   nasal cannula
    b.   nonrebreather mask
    c.   simple face mask
    d.   Venturi mask

60.   When suctioning the upper airway, you should activate the negative pressure:

    a.   when the tip is in the oropharynx
    b.   before insertion
    c.   at the entrance of the mouth
    d.   halfway between the teeth and the pharynx

61.   A patient who is exhibiting wheezing, stridor, accessory muscle use and a weak, ineffective cough is probably suffering from a:

    a.   complete airway obstruction
    b.   partial airway obstruction with good air exchange
    c.   partial airway obstruction with poor air exchange
    d.   none of the above

62.   The proper hand placement position for administering the Heimlich maneuver is:

    a.   between the pubic symphysis and the umbilicus
    b.   just above the umbilicus and well below the xiphoid
    c.   directly over the xiphoid and below the manubrium
    d.   directly over the xiphoid on the midsternum

63. The <u>first step</u> to initiate when a conscious complete airway obstruction victim becomes unconscious is to perform a(n):

     a. abdominal thrust (Heimlich maneuver)
     b. back blow
     c. ventilation
     d. finger sweep

64. All of the following signs are associated with complete upper airway obstruction <u>except</u>:

     a. hand on the throat
     b. inability to speak
     c. absent breath sounds on one side
     d. stridor

65. The most definitive sign of a complete airway obstruction in a conscious person is:

     a. cyanosis of the skin
     b. wheezing on inspiration
     c. snoring on expiration
     d. inability to speak

66. The correct location for a chest thrust to relieve a foreign body obstruction is:

     a. the upper portion of the sternum
     b. the sternum on nipple line
     c. the lower half of the sternum
     d. directly over the xiphoid process

67. If the initial attempt at ventilation is unsuccessful in an unconscious patient, you should next:

     a. deliver four back blows
     b. deliver four abdominal thrusts
     c. reopen the airway and attempt ventilation
     d. perform a finger sweep

68. When encountering a patient with a complete airway obstruction caused by an allergic reaction, you should:

     a. deliver four abdominal thrusts
     b. perform a finger sweep
     c. initiate rapid transport while attempting to ventilate
     d. insert a nasopharyngeal airway to clear the obstruction

69. When attempting to clear a complete airway obstruction in the unconscious patient, you should administer ____ abdominal thrusts.

    a. 2-4
    b. 4-6
    c. 6-10
    d. 2-15

70. In a child or infant with a complete airway obstruction, you should perform a finger sweep only if:

    a. the patient is conscious
    b. the epiglottis is visible
    c. three attempts at ventilation are unsuccessful
    d. you can visualize the object

71. In which of the following patients can back blows be used in the treatment of a complete airway obstruction?

    a. less than 1 year old
    b. 1-8 years old
    c. 8-10 years old
    d. over 10 years old

72. Itching, hives, edema, shortness of breath, wheezing and stridor are all signs of:

    a. foreign body airway obstruction
    b. epiglottitis
    c. croup
    d. anaphylaxis

73. The term "blue bloater" describes what form of chronic obstructive pulmonary disease?

    a. asthma
    b. chronic bronchitis
    c. emphysema
    d. croup

74. The most common breath sound found in patients suffering from an acute asthmatic attack is:

    a. crackles
    b. rhonchi
    c. wheezes
    d. friction rubs

Chapter 3

75.    Patients suffering from emphysema or bronchitis who are pink, alert and
       oriented and ventilating forcefully should receive approximately _____ %
       oxygen.

       a.    21
       b.    24
       c.    75
       d.    90

76.    A patient with asthma, emphysema or bronchitis who is breathing rapidly and
       shallowly at a rate of 32 and who is unresponsive should receive:

       a.    oxygen via nonrebreather mask
       b.    positive pressure ventilation
       c.    oxygen via nasal cannula
       d.    oxygen via Venturi mask

77.    A possible complication of high concentration oxygen administration for a
       chronic obstructive pulmonary disease patient is:

       a.    pneumothorax
       b.    oxygen toxicity
       c.    pneumonia
       d.    respiratory arrest

78.    The patient suffering from chronic obstructive pulmonary disease primarily
       relies upon low blood concentrations of _____ to provide the
       stimulus for breathing.

       a.    carbon dioxide
       b.    oxygen
       c.    hemoglobin
       d.    nitrogen

79.    An inflammation of the alveolar spaces caused by various types of infectious
       organisms or by aspiration of fluid into the tracheobronchial tree is called:

       a.    pneumonia
       b.    pleurisy
       c.    pneumothorax
       d.    pulmonary embolism

80.    Massive pulmonary edema (large amounts of fluid in the lungs) is most
       common in which type of drowning?

       a.    fresh water
       b.    salt water
       c.    dry drowning
       d.    both a and c

81.  Respiratory arrest is most often due to injury or depressant effects upon the:

   a.   cerebrum
   b.   medulla and pons (brainstem)
   c.   cerebellum
   d.   hypothalamus

82.  A condition that results from air entering the pleural space causing total or partial collapse of the lungs is called:

   a.   hemothorax
   b.   pneumothorax
   c.   pleurisy
   d.   hemothorax

83.  When a "sucking" wound is encountered following penetrating chest trauma, the most important treatment for all patients is:

   a.   splinting the chest wall
   b.   immediate positive pressure ventilation
   c.   application of a three-sided airtight dressing
   d.   placing the patient on the nonaffected chest wall

84.  The most common breath sound associated with a pneumothorax is:

   a.   diminished or absent
   b.   wheezes
   c.   rhonchi
   d.   friction rub

85.  A patient with a penetrating chest wound who becomes increasingly short of breath, cyanotic and unresponsive following the application of an airtight dressing and who also exhibits distended neck veins and tracheal shift is probably suffering from:

   a.   pericardial tamponade
   b.   flail chest
   c.   traumatic asphyxia
   d.   tension pneumothorax

86.  If a patient develops an alteration of mental state, tracheal shift and distended neck veins following the application of an airtight dressing to a sucking chest wound, your immediate action should be to:

   a.   temporarily remove the dressing
   b.   provide positive pressure ventilation
   c.   lay the patient on the nonaffected side
   d.   splint the chest wall

87.  The definition of a flail chest is:

 a.  five consecutive broken ribs on the same side
 b.  two or more ribs fractured in two or more places
 c.  a fracture of the sternum and ribs in combination
 d.  open fractures of multiple ribs

88.  The treatment for a flail chest includes:

 a.  an airtight dressing on the affected side
 b.  taping a towel or blanket over the flail segment
 c.  wrapping a dressing around the circumference of the chest
 d.  placing the patient in the prone position

## Case Histories

| Case History #1 |
| --- |
| You are dispatched to a call for difficulty breathing. At the scene, you find a 28 year old female patient who has collapsed on the sidewalk after eating pizza. The patient is pale and complaining of shortness of breath.  Her vital signs are pulse 120/min, blood pressure 70/50 and respirations 32/min.  Her husband states that she is under a doctor's care for a sensitivity to food preservatives. On physical assessment you note that the patient has evidence of hives over her body, is wheezing bilaterally and has stridor on inspiration. |

89.  The most probable cause of her condition is:

 a.  foreign body obstruction
 b.  anaphylaxis
 c.  epiglotitis
 d.  croup

90.  If this patient were to develop a complete airway obstruction, what would be your immediate action?

 a.  deliver abdominal thrusts and attempt to ventilate
 b.  perform a finger sweep and abdominal thrusts
 c.  initiate rapid transport while attempting to ventilate
 d.  insert a nasal pharyngeal airway to clear the obstruction

91. What medication might a patient with this condition carry for self-administration to prevent obstruction of the airway?

    a. epinephrine
    b. orinase
    c. dilantin
    d. Zantac

---

### Case History #2

You are dispatched to a call for difficulty breathing. At the scene, you find a 25 year old female patient lying supine and laboring to breathe. She is exhausted and too breathless to speak. The family advises you that she is being treated for asthma. Her vital signs are pulse 120/min, blood pressure 160/80 and respirations 30/min and shallow. On physical assessment, you note the patient is cyanotic and very sleepy. Her breath sounds are barely audible, and you hear faint wheezing on both sides of the chest.

---

92. The major problem with this patient is:

    a. fluid collecting in the alveoli
    b. narrowing of the bronchioles
    c. swelling of the vocal cords
    d. inflammation of the pleura

93. The initial management of the patient should include:

    a. positive pressure ventilation
    b. administering oxygen via a nasal cannula
    c. sitting the patient up and suctioning the airway
    d. administering oxygen via a simple face mask

---

### Case History #3

Driving while intoxicated, a 35 year old male struck a utility pole. At the scene, you find him still in the driver's seat, unresponsive and laboring to breathe. There is no evidence of facial trauma, and his airway is clear. A quick primary survey reveals that the right anterior chest wall bulges outward on expiration and inward on inspiration. He is actively using his accessory muscles and is cyanotic. His vital signs are pulse 120/min, blood pressure 90/60 and respirations 30/min and shallow.

---

94. What type of chest injury has this patient most likely sustained?

    a. pericardial tamponade
    b. tension pneumothorax
    c. flail chest
    d. traumatic asphyxia

95. Which of the following treatments should be provided to stabilize his condition?

    a.    splinting the chest wall with a towel or blanket
    b.    positive pressure ventilation
    c.    oxygen via nasal cannula
    d.    both a and b

---

### Case History #4

A 32 year old front seat passenger of an automobile collision was just extricated. A bystander states that he was thrown forward against the dashboard. He is in respiratory distress and his vital signs are pulse 120/min, blood pressure 80/50, and respirations are shallow at 36/min. His trachea is deviated to the right and his neck veins are distended. There is subcutaneous emphysema on the upper chest and about the neck. Breath sounds are decreased on the left as compared to the right chest.

---

96. Based on the presenting signs and symptoms, what do you suspect is the underlying condition?

    a.    tension pneumothorax
    b.    flail chest
    c.    pericardial tamponade
    d.    pulmonary embolus

97. The prehospital treatment for this patient would include:

    a.    rapid transport to definitive surgical care
    b.    oxygen via nasal cannula
    c.    splinting the chest wall
    d.    both a and b

98. What definitive intervention is needed at the hospital to temporarily stabilize this patient?

    a.    tracheostomy to secure an airway
    b.    needle decompression of the chest
    c.    needle decompression of the heart
    d.    cricothyroidotomy to secure an airway

---

### Case History #5

You respond to a call for a stabbing. At the scene, you find a 25 year old female who was stabbed in the anterior right chest. The patient is in obvious severe respiratory distress and is exhibiting cyanosis of the lips and nailbeds. Her vital signs are pulse 100/min, blood pressure 110/70, and respirations 26/min. On physical assessment, you note absent breath sounds on the right side of the chest, with blood bubbling from the stab wound.

---

99.   Based on the presentation, what is the underlying condition?

    a.       pulmonary contusion
    b.       flail chest
    c.       pericardial tamponade
    d.       pneumothorax

100.   You apply an airtight dressing and you note that the patient's ventilations appear adequate but she remains cyanotic. What oxygen delivery system would you use on this patient?

    a.       Venturi mask
    b.       nasal cannula
    c.       nonrebreather mask
    d.       simple face mask

101.   After performing the appropriate treatment, the patient does well for about 10 minutes. Then she develops signs of increasing respiratory distress, agitation, and neck vein distention, and her trachea deviates to the left. What would your next immediate action be?

    a.       turn the patient on the noninjured side
    b.       begin positive pressure ventilation
    c.       temporarily remove the dressing
    d.       insert an oropharyngeal airway

---

### Case History #6

You respond to a call for a swimming pool injury. At the scene, you find a 7 year old boy floating supine and slightly submerged in an indoor pool. The patient is unconscious and appears to be cyanotic from the shoulders up. His grandmother (who cannot swim) states that he dove into a shallow part of the pool and did not come up for 2-3 minutes.

---

102.   What major consideration should you exercise during removal from the water?

    a.       a quick abdominal thrust as soon as possible
    b.       spinal immobilization precautions
    c.       beginning compressions in the water
    d.       suctioning prior to ventilation

103. Upon removal, what manual airway maneuver would you use to evaluate breathing?

    a.    head tilt-chin lift
    b.    chin pull maneuver
    c.    head tilt-neck lift
    d.    jaw thrust without head tilt

104. Upon removal you note vital signs are pulse 80/min, blood pressure 80/60, and respirations 2/min. The patient is unresponsive and cyanotic. What breathing rate would you use on this patient?

    a.    1 breath every 3 seconds
    b.    1 breath every 4 seconds
    c.    1 breath every 5 seconds
    d.    1 breath every 7 seconds

---

### Case History #7

A 16 year old boy was found unresponsive and cyanotic in the kitchen by his parents . They say that he was not breathing but had a pulse. They attempted CPR, but there was no response. It has been 4 minutes since they discovered him.

---

105. You open his airway and attempt to ventilate but encounter resistance and observe no chest rise. Your <u>first</u> action should be:

    a.    reopen the airway and attempt to ventilate
    b.    perform a finger sweep maneuver
    c.    apply 6-10 abdominal thrusts
    d.    rapidly transport the patient to the hospital

106. After several maneuvers, you are able to effectively ventilate the patient. What should you do next?

    a.    continue ventilating and transport
    b.    check for a pulse
    c.    suction the airway to ensure patency
    d.    place the patient on his side

107. The correct rescuer position for administering an abdominal thrust is:

    a.    kneeling adjacent but parallel to the patient
    b.    straddling the thighs of the patient
    c.    straddling the umbilicus of the patient
    d.    straddling the lower legs of the patient

---

### Case History #8

You are dispatched to a call for difficulty breathing. At the scene you find a 32 year old female complaining of dizziness and dyspnea. She states that she has been under a lot of stress and just had an argument with her boss. She also complains that she has numbness around her lips and that her fingers and toes feel crampy. Vital signs are pulse 100/min, blood pressure 130/80 and respirations 36/min and very deep. On physical examination, you observe a thin, anxious woman breathing very deeply. Lung fields are clear bilaterally. She has no past history of respiratory conditions.

---

108. Based on the presenting history and physical findings, what would be a likely cause of this patient's signs and symptoms?

    a.  hyperventilation syndrome
    b.  asthma
    c.  emphysema
    d.  pulmonary embolus

109. What is the medical term used to describe the crampy fingers and toes?

    a.  phalanx spasm
    b.  digital spasm
    c.  carpopedal spasm
    d.  metatarsal spasm

110. What is the most important treatment for this patient?

    a.  oxygen via nonrebreather mask
    b.  positive pressure ventilation
    c.  calming reassurance
    d.  rapid transport to the hospital

Skill Performance Sheet

## Inserting an Oropharyngeal Airway

Student Name_____          Date_____

| Performance Standard | Performed | Failed |
|---|---|---|
| Take universal precautions (gloves, goggles) | | |
| Measure airway from mouth to angle of jaw | | |
| Open mouth with cross finger or tongue-jaw lift | | |
| Insert airway with point toward roof of mouth | | |
| Rotate airway when safely past tongue | | |
| Flange rests on outer lips | | |
| Remove airway if gag reflex is noted | | |

Comments_____

_____

_____

_____

Instructor _____          Circle One:   Pass   Fail

Skill Performance Sheet

# Inserting a Nasopharyngeal Airway

Student Name_____          Date_____

| Performance Standard | Performed | Failed |
|---|---|---|
| Take universal precautions (gloves, goggles) | | |
| Measure airway from nares to tip of the ear | | |
| Lubricate airway with surgical jelly | | |
| Insert airway into nasal opening until flange touches opening of nares | | |
| If resistance is encountered, try other nostril | | |

Comments_____

_____

_____

_____

Instructor _____          Circle One:   Pass   Fail

Skill Performance Sheet

# Inserting an Esophageal Gastric Tube Airway

Student Name_____          Date_____

| Performance Standard | Performed | Failed |
|---|---|---|
| Take universal precautions (gloves, goggles) | | |
| Check equipment | | |
| Ensure adequate ventilation with other method prior to insertion | | |
| Place head in neutral or slightly flexed position | | |
| Perform tongue-jaw lift | | |
| Insert tube into posterior pharynx until face mask contacts face | | |
| Seal mask against face and attempt ventilation | | |
| Observe chest rise and auscultate chest and epigastric region | | |
| Inflate cuff with approximately 35 ml of air | | |
| Recheck ventilation | | |

Comments_____

_____

_____

_____

_____

Instructor _____          Circle One:   Pass   Fail

Skill Performance Sheet

# Endotracheal Intubation

Student Name_____          Date_____

| Performance Standard | Performed | Failed |
|---|---|---|
| Take universal precautions (gloves, goggles) | | |
| Check equipment | | |
| Ensure adequate ventilation with other method prior to insertion | | |
| Place head in "sniffing" position | | |
| Hold laryngoscope in left hand | | |
| Insert blade in mouth carefully | | |
| <u>Curved blade:</u>  place blade in vallecula and view epiglottis view glottic opening | | |
| <u>Straight blade:</u>  place blade beyond epiglottis and view glottic opening | | |
| Insert tube cuff slightly beyond vocal cords | | |
| Inflate cuff as appropriate | | |
| Ventilate and auscultate chest and epigastric region | | |
| Insert oropharyngeal airway | | |
| Tape airway and ET tube in place | | |

Comments_____

_____

_____

Instructor _____          Circle One:   Pass   Fail

*Chapter 3*

Skill Performance Sheet

# Mouth to Mouth Breathing

Student Name_____ Date_____

| Performance Standard | Performed | Failed |
|---|---|---|
| Open airway with appropriate maneuver (head tilt-chin lift or jaw thrust) | | |
| Assess breathing (look, listen and feel) | | |
| Seal mouth around the patient's mouth and pinch nose | | |
| Give two smooth breaths while observing chest rise (1-1.5 seconds per breath) | | |
| Take mouth away between breaths | | |
| Check carotid pulse (pulse is present) | | |
| Give one breath every 5 seconds for adult (every 4 for child) | | |

Comments_____

_____

_____

_____

Instructor _____ Circle One:  Pass  Fail

Skill Performance Sheet

# Mouth to Nose Breathing

Student Name_____     Date_____

| Performance Standard | Performed | Failed |
|---|---|---|
| Open airway with appropriate maneuver (head tilt-chin lift or jaw thrust) | \| | \| |
| Assess breathing (look, listen and feel) | \| | \| |
| Seal mouth around the patient's nose and seal mouth | \| | \| |
| Give two smooth breaths while observing chest rise (1-1.5 seconds per breath) | \| | \| |
| Open mouth to allow for exhalation | | \| |
| Check carotid pulse (pulse is present) | \| | \| |
| Give one breath every 5 seconds for an adult (every 4 for child) | \| | \| |

Comments_____

_____

_____

_____

Instructor _____     Circle One:   Pass   Fail

Skill Performance Sheet

# Infant Mouth to Mouth and Nose Breathing

Student Name_____          Date_____

| Performance Standard | Performed | Failed |
| --- | --- | --- |
| Open airway with appropriate maneuver (head tilt-chin lift or jaw thrust) | | |
| Assess breathing (look, listen and feel) | | |
| Seal mouth around the patient's mouth and nose | | |
| Give two smooth breaths while observing chest rise (1-1.5 seconds per breath) | | |
| Take mouth away between breaths | | |
| Check brachial pulse (pulse is present) | | |
| Give one breath every 3 seconds (adult) | | |

Comments_____

_____

_____

_____

Instructor _____          Circle One:  Pass  Fail

Skill Performance Sheet

# Pocket Mask Breathing

Student Name_____          Date_____

| Performance Standard | Performed | Failed |
|---|---|---|
| Take universal precautions (gloves, goggles) | | |
| Check pocket mask before use | | |
| Assess breathing (look, listen and feel) | | |
| Seal mask around patient's mouth with nose portion placed on the bridge of nose | | |
| Maintain seal with two hands and maintain head tilt with fingers along the jaw line | | |
| Give two smooth breaths while observing chest rise | | |
| Give one breath every 5 seconds | | |

Comments_____

_____

_____

_____

Instructor _____          Circle One:   Pass   Fail

Skill Performance Sheet

# Bag-Valve-Mask Breathing

Student Name_____          Date_____

| Performance Standard | Performed | Failed |
|---|---|---|
| Take universal precautions (gloves, goggles) | | |
| Connect reservoir and oxygen | | |
| Check oxygen flow rate | | |
| Check bag-valve-mask before use | | |
| Assess breathing (look, listen and feel) | | |
| Seal mask around patient's mouth with nose portion placed on the bridge of nose | | |
| Maintain seal with C clamp; maintain head tilt with fingers along the jaw line | | |
| Squeeze the bag against the patient's head or your body while observing chest rise | | |
| Give one breath every 5 seconds | | |

Comments_____

_____

_____

_____

Instructor _____          Circle One:   Pass   Fail

Skill Performance Sheet

# Manually Triggered Resuscitator

Student Name_____          Date_____

| Performance Standard | Performed | Failed |
|---|---|---|
| Take universal precautions (gloves, goggles) | | |
| Check resuscitator before use | | |
| Assess breathing (look, listen and feel) | | |
| Seal mask around patient's mouth with nose portion placed on the bridge of nose | | |
| Maintain seal with C clamp; maintain head tilt with fingers along the jaw line | | |
| Push button or squeeze lever while observing chest rise | | |
| Give one breath every 5 seconds | | |

Comments_____

_____

_____

_____

Instructor _____          Circle One:   Pass   Fail

Skill Performance Sheet

# Setting Up an Oxygen System

Student Name_____          Date_____

| Performance Standard | Performed | Failed |
|---|---|---|
| Confirm that gas is oxygen | | |
| Check for rubber washer | | |
| Open main valve to clear opening | | |
| Immediately close valve | | |
| Attach regulator (carefully aligning pin index system) | | |
| Tighten regulator with hand pressure | | |
| Open main valves two full turns | | |
| Check pressure gauge | | |
| Attach delivery device to regulator | | |
| Adjust flow rate | | |
| Attach delivery device to patient | | |

Comments_____

_____

_____

_____

Instructor _____          Circle One:  Pass  Fail

Skill Performance Sheet

# Detaching a Regulator From an Oxygen Cylinder

Student Name_____          Date_____

| Performance Standard | Performed | Failed |
|---|---|---|
| Turn off main valve | | |
| Bleed regulator | | |
| Loosen clamp and detach regulator | | |
| Store in appropriate area | | |

Comments_____

_____

_____

_____

Instructor _____          Circle One:   Pass   Fail

Skill Performance Sheet

# Oropharyngeal Suctioning

Student Name _____     Date _____

| Performance Standard | Performed | Failed |
|---|---|---|
| Take universal precautions (gloves, goggles) | | |
| Test suction device | | |
| Measure catheter from mouth to ear | | |
| Insert catheter or rigid tip in to posterior pharynx | | |
| Apply suction during removal | | |
| Do not exceed 10 seconds | | |

Comments _____

_____

_____

_____

Instructor _____     Circle One:   Pass   Fail

Skill Performance Sheet

# Conscious Complete Airway Obstruction

Student Name_____          Date_____

| Performance Standard | Performed | Failed |
|---|---|---|
| Confirm obstruction by asking "Are you choking?" | | |
| Apply manual abdominal thrusts (chest thrusts for pregnant or obese patient) | | |
| Repeat thrusts until effective or until the patient becomes unconscious | | |

Comments_____

_____

_____

_____

Instructor _____          Circle One:   Pass   Fail

55

Skill Performance Sheet

# Conscious Complete Airway Obstruction That Becomes Unconscious

Student Name_____          Date_____

| Performance Standard | Performed | Failed |
|---|---|---|
| Perform finger sweep (in child only if object is visible) | | |
| Open airway and attempt to ventilate | | |
| Apply 6 to 10 abdominal thrusts | | |
| Perform finger sweep | | |
| Attempt to ventilate | | |
| Repeat sequence of thrusts, finger sweeps and ventilation until effective | | |

Comments_____

_____

_____

_____

Instructor _____          Circle One:  Pass  Fail

Skill Performance Sheet

# Unconscious Complete Airway Obstruction

Student Name_____          Date_____

| Performance Standard | Performed | Failed |
|---|---|---|
| Check for unresponsiveness | | |
| Place the patient in supine position | | |
| Open airway | | |
| Attempt to ventilate (obstructive) | | |
| Perform 6 to 10 abdominal thrusts | | |
| Perform finger sweep | | |
| Attempt to ventilate | | |
| Repeat sequence of thrusts, sweeps and ventilation until effective | | |

Comments_____

_____

_____

_____

Instructor _____          Circle One:   Pass   Fail

*Chapter 4*

## THE CARDIOVASCULAR SYSTEM

1.     The average adult has approximately _____ liters of blood volume.

    a.     1-2
    b.     3-4
    c.     5-6
    d.     7-8

2.     The protein responsible for the transport of oxygen and carbon dioxide is called:

    a.     protoplasm
    b.     platelets
    c.     plasma
    d.     hemoglobin

3.     The cellular portion of the blood that is responsible for combating infection is the:

    a.     platelets
    b.     red blood cells
    c.     white blood cells
    d.     hemoglobin

4.     The portion of blood responsible for clotting is called:

    a.     platelets
    b.     red blood cells
    c.     white blood cells
    d.     plasma

5.     Which of the following blood cells are likely to increase in number during an infection?

    a.     platelets
    b.     red blood cells
    c.     white blood cells
    d.     plasma

6.     The portion of the heart that pumps blood to the body (systemic circulation) is called the:

    a.     left atrium
    b.     right atrium
    c.     left ventricle
    d.     right ventricle

7.  The portion of the heart that receives blood returning from the lungs is called the:

    a.    left atrium
    b.    right atrium
    c.    left ventricle
    d.    right ventricle

8.  The valve that directs blood into the pulmonary artery during systole and prevents backflow into the ventricle during diastole is called the:

    a.    aortic valve
    b.    pulmonary semilunar valve
    c.    tricuspid valve
    d.    mitral valve

9.  The portion of the conduction system that is the primary pacemaker of the heart is called the:

    a.    SA node
    b.    Purkinje fiber
    c.    AV node
    d.    bundle of His

10. The amount of blood ejected from the heart with each contraction is called the:

    a.    cardiac output
    b.    tidal volume
    c.    cardiac reserve
    d.    stroke volume

11. An increase in cardiac output that occurs as a result of an increase in venous return and an increased stretch of the ventricle is a direct result of:

    a.    osmosis
    b.    Starling's law
    c.    oncotic pressure
    d.    diffusion

12. Cardiac output times peripheral vascular resistance (the diameter and tone of the vessels) is the formula that determines:

    a.    stroke volume
    b.    blood pressure
    c.    blood volume
    d.    vital capacity

13. Blood is poor in oxygen and rich in carbon dioxide in all of the following structures except the:

   a. pulmonary artery
   b. vena cava
   c. right ventricle
   d. pulmonary vein

14. Which of the following vessels are most muscular?

   a. arteries
   b. veins
   c. capillaries
   d. venules

15. The systolic pressure best reflects the _____ phase of the cardiac cycle.

   a. contraction
   b. relaxation
   c. intermediate
   d. recovery

16. Gravity, ventilation, valves and muscular activity all contribute to:

   a. increasing oxygen production
   b. venous return
   c. controlling hemorrhage
   d. fighting infections

17. Which of the following vessels contain valves?

   a. arteries
   b. veins
   c. capillaries
   d. arterioles

18. The femoral, popliteal and dorsalis pedis arteries are all located in the:

   a. head
   b. lower extremities
   c. upper extremities
   d. trunk

19. The diastolic pressure best reflects the _____ phase of the cardiac cycle.

   a. contraction
   b. relaxation
   c. intermediate
   d. rapid firing

20. If the cardiac output remained the same and the arteries constricted, the blood pressure would:

    a. remain the same
    b. increase
    c. decrease
    d. none of the above

21. Which of the following is a function of the cardiovascular system?

    a. delivering oxygen and transporting waste for excretion
    b. bringing oxygen into the body from the environment
    c. preparing glucose to enter cells
    d. producing and secreting hormones to regulate body activities

22. The most oxygen dependent organ is the:

    a. heart
    b. intestine
    c. brain
    d. kidney

23. Blood transports most of the body's oxygen via:

    a. plasma
    b. white blood cells
    c. red blood cells
    d. platelets

24. The thin covering of the heart that contains a lubricating fluid is called the:

    a. pleura
    b. peritoneum
    c. mediastinum
    d. pericardium

25. Blood that is poorly saturated with oxygen gives a _____ color to the lips and nailbeds.

    a. pale
    b. pink
    c. blue
    d. cherry red

26. At room air, hemoglobin transports _____ of the oxygen in the blood.

    a. 2%
    b. 50%
    c. 75%
    d. 98%

27.   The superior portion of the heart is located in the upper chest at level of the second rib and is called the:

    a.    apex
    b.    base
    c.    precordium
    d.    apical region

28.   The inferior portion of the heart is located in the left lower chest at level of 5th or 6th rib at mid-clavicular line and is called the:

    a.    apex
    b.    base
    c.    precordium
    d.    apical region

Match the layer of the heart in column A with the description in column B.

| Column A | | Column B | |
| --- | --- | --- | --- |
| 29. | myocardium | a. | smooth inner lining |
| 30. | epicardium | b. | outermost layer |
| 31. | endocardium | c. | thick muscular layer |

32.   The upper receiving chambers of the heart are called the:

    a.    ventricles
    b.    septum
    c.    atria
    d.    pleura

33.   The wall that separates the left and right sides of the heart is called the:

    a.    ventricles
    b.    septum
    c.    atria
    d.    pleura

34.   The left circulation is the _____ circulation.

    a.    pulmonary
    b.    systemic
    c.    arterial
    d.    venous

35. The right circulation is the _____ circulation.

    a. pulmonary
    b. systemic
    c. arterial
    d. venous

36. The valves that control flow from the atria to the ventricles are the _____ valves.

    a. semilunar
    b. atrioventricular
    c. atrial
    d. ventricular

37. The valves that control flow from the ventricles to the pulmonary arteries and aorta are the _____ valves.

    a. semilunar
    b. atrioventricular
    c. atrial
    d. ventricular

38. The amount of blood ejected from the ventricle with each contraction is called the:

    a. stroke volume
    b. cardiac output
    c. pulmonary flow
    d. tidal volume

39. Cardiac output is the stroke volume multiplied by the average _____ per minute.

    a. tidal volume
    b. heart rate
    c. respiratory rate
    d. vital capacity

40. The first arteries to branch off the aorta and supply blood to the heart are called the _____ arteries.

    a. systemic
    b. brachial
    c. coronary
    d. pulmonary

41.    Gas exchange occurs in which of the following vessels?

    a.    arteries
    b.    veins
    c.    capillaries
    d.    venules

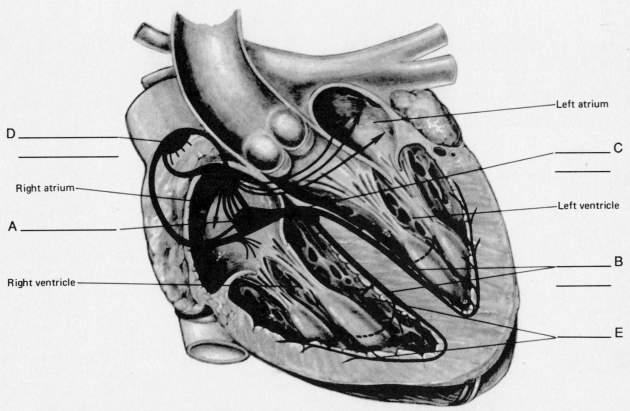

(Solomon EP, Phillips GA:  Understanding Human Anatomy and Physiology.  Philadelphia, WB Saunders, 1987, p 214)

Match the terms below with the diagram of the conduction system above.

C 42.    bundle branches          D 45.    SA node (pacemaker)

a 43.    AV node                      C 46.    bundle of His

E 44.    Purkinje fibers

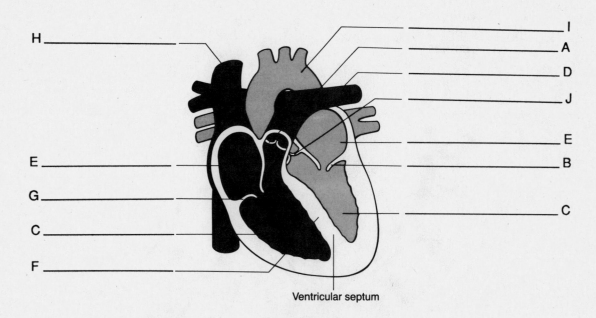

Ventricular septum

Match the terms below with the diagram of the heart above.

*B* 47.  mitral valve      *C* 52.  ventricle

*F* 48.  septum      *A* 53.  pulmonary semilunar valve

*E* 49.  atrium      *D* 54.  pulmonary artery

*G* 50.  tricuspid valve      *J* 55.  aortic semilunar valve

*I* 51.  aorta      *H* 56.  vena cava

57.  Movement of particles from an area of higher concentration to an area of lower concentration best describes:

     a.  diffusion
     b.  osmosis
     c.  oncotic pressure
     d.  Starling's Law

58.  The movement of water from an area of lower concentration of particles to an area of higher concentration of particles best describes:

     a.  diffusion
     b.  osmosis
     c.  oncotic pressure
     d.  Starling's law

59.    The rate and force of contraction of the heart is regulated through the
_____ nervous system

    a.    peripheral
    b.    autonomic
    c.    voluntary
    d.    general

60.    An increase in parasympathetic tone within the nervous system will result in
which of the following responses?

    a.    the pulse will increase
    b.    the force of contraction will increase
    c.    the pulse will slow
    d.    the force of contraction will decrease

## Chapter 5

## CARDIOVASCULAR EMERGENCIES

1.  Failure of the circulatory system to adequately perfuse and oxygenate the tissues of the body best defines:

    a. respiratory failure
    b. shock
    c. heart failure
    d. clinical death

2.  The "fight or flight" response is mediated by:

    a. atropine
    b. epinephrine
    c. histamine
    d. dopamine

3.  Which of the following is an effect of adrenaline release?

    a. decreased heart rate
    b. constriction of the pupils
    c. increased force of heart contraction
    d. decreased flow to the brain

4.  Gravity, muscles and valves, and inspiration and expiration are all forces directly influencing:

    a. stroke volume
    b. heart rate
    c. venous return
    d. coronary artery blood flow

5.  During shock, organs are perfused preferentially by the redistribution of blood. Which organ is the last to be perfused?

    a. heart
    b. kidneys
    c. lungs
    d. brain

6.  Shock that occurs secondary to a myocardial infarction (heart attack) is called:

    a. cardiogenic shock
    b. distributive shock
    c. obstructive shock
    d. hypovolemic shock

7.    Which of the following is most likely to result in vasodilatory type shock?

    a.    anaphylaxis
    b.    hemorrhage
    c.    tension pneumothorax
    d.    heart attack

8.    Which of the following conditions may cause obstructive shock?

    a.    coronary thrombosis
    b.    anaphylaxis
    c.    myocardial infarction
    d.    tension pneumothorax

9.    Which of the following conditions may cause hypovolemic shock?

    a.    diarrhea
    b.    burns
    c.    vomiting
    d.    all of the above

10.   A condition characterized by a low supply of hemoglobin is:

    a.    hypotensive syndrome
    b.    anemia
    c.    ischemia
    d.    hypovolemia

11.   Bleeding characterized by pulsatile flow and bright red blood is:

    a.    capillary
    b.    venous
    c.    systemic
    d.    arterial

12.   Which of the following is a characteristic of venous bleeding?

    a.    pulsatile flow
    b.    dark red color
    c.    occurs in deep wounds
    d.    always requires pressure point to control

13.   The first step used to control bleeding is:

    a.    pressure point
    b.    tourniquet
    c.    air splint
    d.    direct pressure

14. Which of the following steps of bleeding control should be done as the final method?

    a. direct pressure
    b. tourniquet
    c. pressure point
    d. elevation

15. The pressure point for the upper extremity is located over the:

    a. femoral artery
    b. radial artery
    c. ulna artery
    d. brachial artery

16. The pressure point for the lower extremity is located over the:

    a. femoral artery
    b. radial artery
    c. ulna artery
    d. brachial artery

17. The pressure point for the scalp is located over the:

    a. carotid artery
    b. facial artery
    c. temporal artery
    d. brachial artery

18. Which of the following is a possible complication of lacerated vein in the neck or upper chest?

    a. air embolism
    b. pneumothorax
    c. hemothorax
    d. tissue necrosis

19. Orthostatic hypotension is best described as a <u>minimal</u> blood pressure drop of ___mm Hg when a patient is placed upright.

    a. 5
    b. 10
    c. 20
    d. 40

20. The first compensatory response of the body to acute blood loss (less than 15%) is:

    a. venous constriction
    b. hypotension
    c. arterial constriction
    d. none of the above

21.    Which of the following signs is the last to occur following acute blood loss?

      a.    pale skin
      b.    tachycardia
      c.    delayed capillary refill
      d.    hypotension

22.    Pulse rate increase, delayed capillary refill and orthostatic hypotension usually <u>first</u> appear when blood loss exceeds:

      a.    5%
      b.    10%
      c.    15%
      d.    30%

23.    Which of the following best describes the sequence of the signs of hypovolemic shock?

      a.    coma, rapid pulse, hypotension, delayed capillary refill
      b.    hypotension, rapid pulse, delayed capillary refill, coma
      c.    delayed capillary refill, rapid pulse, hypotension, coma
      d.    rapid pulse, coma, hypotension, delayed capillary refill

24.    Use of the abdominal section of the pneumatic antishock garment (PSAG) is contraindicated in the presence of:

      a.    abdominal evisceration
      b.    suspected ruptured spleen
      c.    contusions on the abdominal wall
      d.    kidney injuries

25.    The PSAG is used in the prehospital treatment of all of the following forms of shock except:

      a.    cardiogenic shock
      b.    distributive shock
      c.    obstructive shock
      d.    hypovolemic shock

26.    When removing the PSAG in the hospital, the blood pressure should never drop by more than _____ mm Hg.

      a.    2
      b.    5
      c.    10
      d.    20

27. Which of the following is a possible effect of the PSAG?

    a. increases peripheral vascular resistance
    b. tamponades bleeding in the chest
    c. transfuses large amounts of blood to torso
    d. shunts blood to the extremities

28. The upper margin of the abdominal section of the PASG should be placed no higher than the:

    a. umbilicus
    b. iliac crest of the pelvis
    c. lower margin of the rib cage
    d. suprapubic region

29. Which of the following is a contraindication to the use of the PSAG?

    a. intraabdominal bleeding
    b. head injury
    c. extremity bleeding
    d. pulmonary edema

30. The leading cause of death in the United States is _____ and its resulting complications.

    a. cancer
    b. accidental death
    c. arteriosclerotic heart disease
    d. AIDS

31. The progressive narrowing of vessels due to plaque formation on the inner most lining best describes:

    a. angioedema
    b. arteriosclerosis
    c. angina pectoris
    d. ischemia

32. A myocardial infarction patient who is demonstrating generalized signs of hypoxia (i.e., cyanosis or altered mental state) and severe chest pain should receive oxygen via a:

    a. nasal cannula
    b. nonrebreather mask
    c. simple face mask
    d. Venturi mask

33. All of the following are major <u>avoidable</u> risk factors of coronary artery disease except:

    a. smoking
    b. alcohol use
    c. hypertension
    d. high blood cholesterol

34. All of the following are methods through which patients take nitroglycerin <u>except</u>:

    a. swallow tablets
    b. inject into muscles
    c. apply paste to skin
    d. place under tongue

35. An insufficient supply of blood through a vessel that results in oxygen deprivation to tissue best describes:

    a. ischemia
    b. hypoxia
    c. anoxia
    d. anemia

36. Blockage of a coronary artery resulting in death of heart tissue defines:

    a. coronary insufficiency
    b. myocardial infarction
    c. angina pectoris
    d. cardiac arrest

37. Nausea, vomiting, weakness, shortness of breath, palpitations, light-headedness, sweating, dizziness and loss of consciousness are all possible associated signs of:

    a. cardiac arrest
    b. angina pectoris
    c. myocardial infarction
    d. oxygen toxicity

38. Chest pain brought on by emotional or physical exertion and relieved by rest best describes:

    a. pleuritic chest pain
    b. angina pectoris
    c. myocardial infarction
    d. cardiogenic shock

39.     The patient should be questioned about high blood pressure, heart disease, chronic obstructive pulmonary disease (COPD) and diabetes during the _____ phase of the history.

   a.     chief complaint
   b.     history of present illness
   c.     medications and allergies
   d.     past medical history

40.     Most persons who die of coronary artery disease die because of:

   a.     pump failure
   b.     arrythmias
   c.     obstructive shock
   d.     valve failure

41.     Nitroglycerin acts to relieve chest pain by which of the following mechanisms?

   a.     increases heart rate
   b.     increases the force of contraction
   c.     causes vasodilation
   d.     increases blood pressure

42.     The symptom that is <u>always</u> present in cases of myocardial infarction is:

   a.     nausea
   b.     chest pain
   c.     shortness of breath
   d.     no symptom is always present

43.     Which of the following terms best describes the <u>classic</u> pain of coronary artery disease, such as angina or myocardial infarction?

   a.     sharp
   b.     squeezing
   c.     pleuritic
   d.     stabbing

44.     The pulse of a patient suffering a myocardial infarction is usually:

   a.     rapid
   b.     almost any variation
   c.     slow
   d.     irregular

45.  Decreasing anxiety, activity and sources of fear is a method for:

  a.  increasing oxygen delivery
  b.  decreasing oxygen demand
  c.  increasing adrenaline release
  d.  dilating coronary arteries

46.  A common reaction to serious illness, including myocardial infarction, that often causes the patient to not seek help is referred to as:

  a.  rationalization
  b.  denial
  c.  confabulation
  d.  anxiety syndrome

47.  Myocardial infarction patients who are experiencing shortness of breath usually prefer to be placed in a _____ position.

  a.  sitting
  b.  supine
  c.  prone
  d.  lateral recumbent

48.  Patients who take nitroglycerin may commonly experience which of the following side effects:

  a.  hives
  b.  arrhythmias
  c.  headache
  d.  edema

49.  The two most important factors in the treatment of <u>cardiac arrest</u> are CPR and:

  a.  defibrillation
  b.  drug therapy
  c.  intubation
  d.  catheterization

Match the the type of heart failure in column B with the signs and symptoms in column A.

| Column A | | Column B | |
| --- | --- | --- | --- |
| *b* 50. | rales | a. | right-sided heart failure |
| *a* 51. | ankle edema | b. | left-sided heart failure |
| *b* 52. | frothy sputum | | |
| *a* 53. | distended neck veins | | |
| *a* 54. | ascites | | |

55. All of the following are typical historical facts that a congestive heart failure patient might describe except:

    a.    sleeps on more than one pillow
    b.    chronic ankle edema
    c.    chest pain on exertion
    d.    wakes up with dyspnea during night

56. When patients with a recent onset of the symptoms of myocardial infarction have severe ankle edema it most likely suggests:

    a.    preexisting heart failure
    b.    cardiogenic shock
    c.    hypertension
    d.    left ventricular failure

57. A condition associated with heart failure that is characterized by waking up in the middle of the night with difficulty breathing is called:

    a.    paroxysmal nocturnal dyspnea
    b.    sleep dyspnea
    c.    supine dyspnea
    d.    bradypnea

58. A condition characterized by difficulty breathing while in the supine position is called:

    a.    eupnea
    b.    tachypnea
    c.    orthopnea
    d.    supnea

59.    The most common cause of cardiogenic shock is:

    a.    chronic obstructive pulmonary disease
    b.    angina
    c.    acute myocardial infarction
    d.    valvular disease

60.    The ventricle cannot pump out an adequate amount of blood and blood backs up through the atria and venous system.  This best describes:

    a.    hypovolemia
    b.    obstructive shock
    c.    heart failure
    d.    distributive shock

61.    The most common cause of right heart failure is

    a.    COPD
    b.    valvular disease
    c.    preexisting left-sided heart failure
    d.    pulmonary embolism

62.    Where is edema most likely to occur <u>first</u> when a patient develops heart failure?

    a.    sacral area
    b.    tibia
    c.    abdomen
    d.    ankles

63.    Fine crackling breath sounds similar to what is heard when rolling pieces of your hair between your fingers next to your ear are called:

    a.    wheezes
    b.    stridor
    c.    rales
    d.    friction rub

64.    A patient with acute pulmonary edema who is becoming sleepy, and cyanotic and who has barely perceptible chest wall movement should be treated with supplemental oxygen via a:

    a.    Ventuir mask
    b.    bag valve mask
    c.    nasal cannula
    d.    simple face mask

65.   Signs of shock in the presence of ischemic chest pain is most likely:

    a.    distributive shock
    b.    obstructive shock
    c.    cardiogenic shock
    d.    hypovolemic shock

66.   An aneurysm caused by blood entering the wall of the aorta with continued leaking along the lining of the inner and middle walls is called a _____ aneurysm.

    a.    berry
    b.    dissecting
    c.    penetrating
    d.    subarachnoid

67.   Sudden onset of unilateral pleuritic chest pain, dyspnea associated with a cough and hemoptysis in a patient with a history of phlebitis and unilateral leg swelling is probably related to:

    a.    angina
    b.    myocardial infarction
    c.    pulmonary embolus
    d.    aneurysm

68.   The term used to describe a slow heart rate (less than 60/min) is:

    a.    bradycardia
    b.    tachycardia
    c.    hypocardia
    d.    hypercardia

69.   Very rapid heart rates may cause decreased cardiac output due to a shortened:

    a.    contraction
    b.    relaxation period (diastole)
    c.    atrial contraction
    d.    depolarization

70.   A sensation that may described as an extra beat skipping, jumping in the chest or runaway heart is called:

    a.    flutterings
    b.    palpitations
    c.    cardia spasms
    d.    undulations

71.    Bleeding into the sac surrounding the heart is commonly called pericardial:

    a.    tamponade
    b.    effusion
    c.    contusion
    d.    hemorrhage

## Case Histories

| Case History #1 |
| --- |
| You respond to a call and find a 26 year old male who was struck by an auto. The primary survey reveals that the patient is alert and oriented, is breathing and has a carotid pulse. He has a wound on his right thigh that is spurting bright red blood. You attempt to control the bleeding with direct pressure and elevation but are unsuccessful. |

72.    Based on the description above the bleeding is most likely:

    a.    venous
    b.    capillary
    c.    arterial
    d.    venule

73.    Your next action is to:

    a.    apply a tourniquet between the wound and heart
    b.    apply a pressure point over the popliteal artery
    c.    clamp the vessel with a hemostat
    d.    apply a pressure point over the femoral artery

74.    If the above action is not successful, then and only then should you:

    a.    apply a tourniquet between the wound and heart
    b.    apply a pressure point over the popliteal artery
    c.    clamp the vessel with a hemostat
    d.    apply a pressure point over the femoral artery

| Case History #2 |
| --- |
| You respond to a call and find a 32 year old female who is the driver of a car involved a front-end collision. She is alert and oriented and appears pale and sweaty with delayed capillary refill; her neck veins are flat. She is complaining of pain in her upper left quadrant of her abdomen and contusions on the left chest and abdominal walls. Her vital signs are respirations 26 and shallow, pulse 120 and regular (at the carotids), and she has no palpable radial pulses. |

75. Based on the above signs you suspect internal blood loss of approximately
    _____ %.

    a.  less than 10
    b.  10-15
    c.  15-20
    d.  greater than 30

76. The absent radial pulses in both arms is probably related to:

    a.  fractures
    b.  low blood pressure
    c.  blood clots
    d.  severed arteries in the arms

77. Based on these findings, which of the following oxygen delivery methods is
    appropriate?

    a.  Venturi mask
    b.  nasal cannula
    c.  simple face mask
    d.  nonrebreather mask

78. Based on the status of the patient, the PASG is:

    a.  not indicated
    b.  indicated
    c.  indicated but for the legs only
    d.  indicated but for the abdominal section only

79. If this patient had grossly distended neck veins, which of the following
    conditions would you search for?

    a.  cardiac contusion
    b.  tension pneumothorax
    c.  aortic aneurysm
    d.  arrhythmias

---

### Case History #3

You respond to a call and find a 30 year old male who fainted after being robbed
at gunpoint. His friend explains that during the stickup the patient fell
unconscious for about one minute. The patient is now alert and oriented and has
a perfectly normal physical exam. His vital signs are pulse 80 and regular, blood
pressure 100/80, and respirations 18 and of normal depth.

---

80. This patient most likely suffered a transient form of _____ shock.

    a.     obstructive
    b.     vasodilatory
    c.     hypovolemic
    d.     cardiogenic

81. What action should his friend have taken to facilitate his recovery?

    a.     sit the patient up
    b.     administer amonia capsules
    c.     elevate his legs while supine
    d.     administer glucose by mouth

82. This patient's primary cardiovascular problem was related to:

    a.     decreased peripheral resistance
    b.     tachycardia
    c.     vasoconstriction of the brain vessels
    d.     obstruction of blood flow through vessels

---

**Case History #4**

A 55 year old male suffers severe pressure like chest pain after walking up 2 flights of stairs. After taking 3 nitroglycerin tablets, his pain subsides 5 minutes following the start of the episode. He tells you that the pain usually subsides after administration of 1 nitroglycerin tablet. He is pale, cool and sweaty. His vital signs are pulse 100 and regular, respirations 20 and normal, and blood pressure 160/90. He is also complaining of a headache. The patient tells you that this happens often and he refuses to go to the hospital.

---

83. The most likely diagnosis for this patient is:

    a.     heart failure
    b.     cardiac syncope
    c.     cardiogenic shock
    d.     angina pectoris

84. The headache that this patient is experiencing is most likely the result of:

    a.     poor brain perfusion due to the heart condition
    b.     high blood pressure
    c.     nitroglycerin administration
    d.     radiation of the chest pain

85.   The reason that this patient must be urged to go to hospital is his:

    a.   malignant hypertension
    b.   poor brain perfusion
    c.   sweaty skin
    (d.)   changing pattern of disease

86.   The pale, cool and sweaty skin is most likely a function of:

    a.   heart failure
    (b.)   adrenaline release
    c.   parasympathetic discharge
    d.   hypertension

87.   If the pain had continued for 20 minutes, your most likely diagnosis would be:

    a.   angina pectoris
    (b.)   myocardial infarction
    c.   cardiogenic shock
    d.   heart failure

---

### Case History #5

You respond to a call and find a 62 year old female complaining of crushing chest pain for 1 hour with pale, sweaty skin. She states that the pain radiates to her left arm and she also feels nausea and dizziness. Upon physical examination, you note vital signs: pulse 110 and very irregular, blood pressure 160/100, and respiration 28 and slightly labored. She has no visible neck vein distention or edema, and her lungs are clear. Her past medical history includes hypertension, diabetes, and emphysema, and her medications are Aldomet and Diabinase. She is allergic to penicillin.

---

88.   The most likely diagnosis for this patient is:

    a.   angina pectoris
    b.   congestive heart failure
    c.   cardiogenic shock
    (d.)   myocardial infarction

89.   What is the most common cause of death related to this condition?

    a.   shock
    (b.)   ventricular fibrillation
    c.   pulmonary edema
    d.   respiratory failure

90. The cause of this condition is:

    a. poor circulation caused by arrhythmias
    b. blockage of a coronary artery
    c. overstretching of the ventricle
    d. bleeding into the arterial wall

---

### Case History #6

You respond to a call and find a 72 year old female complaining of severe shortness of breath. She is sitting upright, is pale and sweaty with cyanotic lips and is actively using her accessory muscles. Upon physical examination, you find grossly distended neck veins, rales throughout her lung fields and frothy red sputum exuding from her mouth. Her abdomen is grossly distended, and she has severe ankle edema. Her vital signs are pulse 110 and regular, blood pressure 190/100, and respirations 30 and labored. She is alert but extremely agitated. She has no history of chronic obstructive pulmonary disease (COPD).

---

91. The most likely diagnosis for this patient is:

    a. congestive heart failure with acute pulmonary edema
    b. myocardial infarction with cardiogenic shock
    c. pulmonary embolism with obstructive shock
    d. acute pulmonary pneumonia

92. The rales are a primary indication of poor function of her:

    a. left atrium
    b. left ventricle
    c. right atrium
    d. right ventricle

93. The distended neck veins, abdominal distention and ankle edema are indicators of poor function of her:

    a. left atrium
    b. left ventricle
    c. right atrium
    d. right ventricle

94. Given the fact that she is alert, agitated and ventilating forcefully, the oxygen device of choice for this patient is:

    a. Venturi mask
    b. bag-valve-mask
    c. nasal cannula
    d. nonrebreather mask

95.    The frothy sputum exuding from this patient's mouth is primarily due to:

     a.     increased mucus production in the lungs
     b.     fluid from the pulmonary capillaries
     c.     infectious secretions within the airway
     d.     vomitus mixed with air

96.    Suddenly the patient becomes lethargic and lies down on the stretcher. Her respiratory rate drops to 9, and she has cyanosis throughout her face. Your first action should be to:

     a.     sit the patient upright to reduce venous return
     b.     place the patient on her side to remove secretions
     c.     begin positive pressure breathing
     d.     increase oxygen via her freeflow device

97.    The cyanosis in this patient is most likely due to:

     a.     poor cardiac output
     b.     poor diffusion at tissues
     c.     poor oxygen diffusion at the alveoli
     d.     decreased hemoglobin

98.    The sleepy lethargic mental state is probably the result of:

     a.     the effects of oxygen therapy
     b.     brain edema
     c.     the effects of cardiac medications
     d.     brain hypoxia

*Chapter 5*

## Skill Performance Sheet

### Bleeding Control

Student Name_____     Date_____

| Performance Standard | Performed | Failed |
|---|---|---|
| Takes universal precautions (gloves, goggles) | | |
| Applies direct pressure | | |
| Elevates extremity | | |
| If bleeding not controlled, applies pressure at correct pressure point | | |
| If bleeding not controlled, applies a tourniquet: | | |
| Selects appropriate material | | |
| Wraps tourniquet around extremity | | |
| Places and secures dowel stick | | |
| Tightens tourniquet until bleeding is controlled | | |
| Marks patient in visible location to document application | | |

Comments_____

_____

_____

_____

Instructor _____     Circle One:  Pass   Fail

Skill Performance Sheet

**Application of the Pneumatic Antishock Garment**

Student Name_____          Date_____

| Performance Standard | Performed | Failed |
|---|---|---|
| States indications for PSAG | | |
| States contraindications for PASG | | |
| Applies garment without compromising spinal injury | | |
| Positions garment properly | | |
| Closes Velcro on abdominal and leg sections | | |
| Inflates all three sections | | |
| Assesses patient response | | |

Comments_____

_____

_____

_____

Instructor _____          Circle One:   Pass   Fail

## Chapter 6

### CPR AND EMT DEFIBRILLATION

1.  The currently recommended procedure for opening the airway of an unconscious patient is the:

    a. head tilt-chin lift
    b. tongue pull
    c. chin pull
    d. triple airway maneuver

2.  The airway maneuver of choice when dealing with a patient with a suspected cervical spine patient is:

    a. jaw thrust without head tilt
    b. chin pull maneuver
    c. head tilt-neck lift
    d. head tilt-chin lift

3.  The best indicator of an effective positive pressure ventilation is:

    a. exhalation sounds
    b. pinking of the skin
    c. chest rise
    d. increase in the pulse rate

4.  Each breath should take approximately _____ seconds to deliver effective volumes of air and avoid gastric distention.

    a. 0.5-1.0
    b. 1.0-1.5
    c. 2.0-3.0
    d. 4.0-5.0

5.  The volume of air required to effectively ventilate a nonbreathing adult is approximately _____ ml.

    a. 250-500
    b. 500-700
    c. 800-1200
    d. 2000-3000

6.  Ventilations for an adult respiratory arrest victim should be provided at a rate of 1 breath every ____ seconds.

    a. 3
    b. 4
    c. 5
    d. 10

7.    If you encounter resistance to your initial ventilation, you should:

    a.    reopen the airway and attempt to ventilate again
    b.    ventilate more forcefully
    c.    provide an abdominal thrust immediately
    d.    check for a pulse

8.    The correct ratio of compressions to ventilations for one-rescuer adult CPR is:

    a.    15:2
    b.    5:1
    c.    15:4
    d.    5:2

9.    The correct ratio of compressions to ventilations for two-rescuer adult CPR is:

    a.    15:2
    b.    5:1
    c.    15:4
    d.    5:2

10.    The correct compression rate for one- and two-rescuer CPR is _____ compressions per minute.

    a.    40-80
    b.    60-90
    c.    80-100
    d.    100-120

11.    The correct depth of compression in an adult patient is approximately:

    a.    1/2 to 1 inch
    b.    1 to 1 1/2 inches
    c.    1 1/2 to 2 inches
    d.    2 to 3 inches

12.    The most likely cause of gastric distention is:

    a.    overcompressions
    b.    abdominal bleeding
    c.    heart failure
    d.    too forceful ventilations

13.     To ensure maximum blood flow during compressions, the compression relaxation ratio should be ____% compression to____% relaxation.

    a.    20/80
    b.    30/70
    c.    40/60
    d.    50/50

14.     During the performance of compressions, you hear a rib break. Your action should be to:

    a.    discontinue compressions
    b.    reassess your compression technique and continue
    c.    compress at a slower rate
    d.    have someone else perform compressions

15.     The point at which pulse and breathing stop is referred to as:

    a.    biological death
    b.    irreversible death
    c.    temporary death
    d.    clinical death

16.     When initially checking the pulse of an unconscious person, you should check for approximately _____ seconds to avoid the missing a slow or weak pulse.

    a.    2-3
    b.    3-5
    c.    5-10
    d.    10-15

17.     To locate the correct position for compressions, you should initially locate the _____ with the fingers of the hand closer to the patient's feet.

    a.    lower margin of the ribcage
    b.    suprasternal notch
    c.    manubrium of the sternum
    d.    left sternal border

18.     Most cardiac arrests in children over 1 year old are a result of:

    a.    accidents or respiratory problems
    b.    coronary artery disease
    c.    genetic defects
    d.    arrhythmias

19. For the purposes of CPR, a child is defined as someone:

    a. newborn to 5 years old
    b. newborn to 3 years old
    c. 1 to 8 years old
    d. 1 to 12 years old

20. When opening the airway of an infant you should:

    a. slightly extend the neck
    b. hyperextend the neck
    c. flex the neck
    d. flex to 90 degrees

21. Ventilation for the infant is provided mouth to:

    a. mouth
    b. nose
    c. mouth and nose
    d. stoma

22. During the assessment phase of CPR, the pulse of an infant is felt over the:

    a. carotid artery
    b. femoral artery
    c. brachial artery
    d. radial artery

23. Ventilations for an infant arrest victim should be provided at a rate of 1 breath every ____ seconds.

    a. 3
    b. 4
    c. 5
    d. 10

24. Chest compressions for the infant are initiated with the tips of two fingers at which of the following locations:

    a. lower half of the sternum
    b. 1 fingerbreadth below nipple line
    c. just below the suprasternal notch
    d. just above the xiphoid process

25. The correct depth of compression for the infant is:

    a. 1/2 to 1 inch
    b. 1/2 to 2 inches
    c. 1 to 1 1/2 inches
    d. 1 1/2 to 2 inches

26.    The correct rate of compression for an infant is _____ compressions per minute.

    a.    60-80
    b.    80-100
    c.    100
    d.    120

27.    The correct ratio of compressions to ventilations for infant CPR is:

    a.    15:2
    b.    5:1
    c.    15:4
    d.    5:2

28.    Ventilations for a child respiratory arrest victim should be provided at a rate of 1 breath every _____ seconds.

    a.    3
    b.    4
    c.    5
    d.    10

29.    The correct depth of compression for the child is:

    a.    1/2 to 1 inch
    b.    1/2 to 2 inches
    c.    1 to 1 1/2 inches
    d.    1 1/2 to 2 inches

30.    The correct rate of compression for an child is _____ compressions per minute.

    a.    60-80
    b.    80-100
    c.    100
    d.    120

31.    The correct ratio of compressions to ventilations for child CPR is:

    a.    15:2
    b.    5:1
    c.    15:4
    d.    5:2

32.    When performing compressions on a child you should use one hand:

    a.    on the lower half of the sternum
    b.    on the upper half of the sternum
    c.    on the nipple line
    d.    just above the nipple line

33.  While performing compressions on a child, you should _____ with the hand closer to the child's head.

   a.  check the pulse
   b.  maintain an open airway
   c.  provide pressure on the cricoid
   d.  monitor your compression position

34.  In which of the following circumstances can CPR be discontinued?

   a.  when the rescuer is too exhausted to continue
   b.  when the patients pupils are constricted
   c.  when the patient becomes pink
   d.  when a rescuer breaks a rib during compressions

35.  The physiologic response that directs blood flow to vital organs in a drowning victim is called the:

   a.  cell preservation response
   b.  dormant response
   c.  mammalian diving reflex
   d.  hibernation reflex

36.  Water in the stomach following a near drowning should be:

   a.  suctioned out with a long catheter
   b.  left alone unless it interferes with ventilation efforts
   c.  removed by a "breaking" maneuver
   d.  removed by applying a chest thrust

37.  Besides the prompt application of CPR, what variables will most affect the survival of a cardiac arrest patient?

   a.  the size of the heart attack
   b.  time to advanced life support (i.e., defibrillation)
   c.  the ventilation device utilized during CPR
   d.  the compression rate

38.  The chaotic electrical rhythm that causes sudden clinical death in most cardiac arrest patients develop is called:

   a.  ventricular asystole
   b.  ventricular fibrillation
   c.  ventricular tachycardia
   d.  ventricular standstill

39.     The origin of prehospital defibrillation dates back to the:

        a:      1940s
        b.      1950s
        c.      1960s
        d.      1970s

Match the electrical and mechanical events in column B to the wave in column A.

| Column A | Column B |
| --- | --- |
| *b* 40.   P wave | a.      ventricles repolarize, no mechanical event |
| *c* 41.   QRS | b.      atria depolarize and contract |
| *a* 42.   T wave | c.      ventricles depolarize and contract |

43.     The rate of discharge of the SA node or pacemaker for an adult is approximately _____ beats per minute.

        a.      20-40
        b.      60-80
        c.      100-120
        d.      140-160

Match the definition in column B with the correct term in column A.

| Column A | Column B |
| --- | --- |
| *b* 44.   automaticity | a.      change in electric potential across a cell membrane that leads to contraction |
| *a* 45.   depolarization | b.      ability of a cell to generate an electrical impulse |
| *c* 46.   conductivity | c.      ability of the heart cell to receive a stimulus from a neighboring cell and pass it on |
| *d* 47.   repolarization | d.      recharging of the cell membrane to its original "polarized" state. |

48. Immediately following contraction, the heart cells enter a(n) _____ period during which they cannot be depolarized.

    a.    excitation
    b.    refractory
    c.    interlude
    d.    stimulation

49. The first part of the conduction system to recharge or repolarize is the:

    a.    SA node (pacemaker)
    b.    AV node
    c.    bundle of His
    d.    Purkinje fibers

50. If the SA node or pacemaker fails, the AV node can initiate contractions at a rate of _____ per minute.

    a.    20-40
    b.    40-60
    c.    60-80
    d.    80-100

51. If the SA node and AV node fail, the ventricles can initiate contractions at a rate of _____ per minute.

    a.    20-40
    b.    40-60
    c.    60-80
    d.    80-100

52. The electrical activity of the heart is commonly measured by an instrument that detects and amplifies the electrical signals called the:

    a.    defibrillator
    b.    electrocardiogram
    c.    electroencephalogram
    d.    electrograph

53. An ECG machine is connected to the body's surface by_____ and cables.

    a.    electrodes
    b.    interfacers
    c.    connection modules
    d.    none of the above

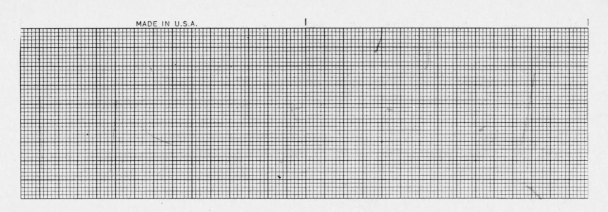

54. The dark vertical markings on the EKG paper correspond to ____ seconds in time.

    a. 0.1
    b. 0.2
    c. 0.3
    d. 0.5

Match the time in seconds in column B with the related number of dark vertical lines on an EKG tracing in column A.

| Column A | | Column B | |
|---|---|---|---|
| 55. | 5 lines | a. | 0.6 seconds |
| 56. | 3 lines | b. | 1.0 seconds |
| 57. | 10 lines | c. | 4.0 seconds |
| 58. | 20 lines | d. | 2.0 seconds |

59. The periodic marks that measure time marks on the top of most types of ECG paper appear every _____ seconds.

    a. 1
    b. 2
    c. 3
    d. 5

60. By counting the number of ventricular complexes within 2 top periodic markings on EKG paper and multiplying times ___, you can estimate the EKG rate.

    a. 2
    b. 3
    c. 5
    d. 10

61. Standardization is usually calibrated so that a ____ mm deflection (10 small boxes on the EKG paper) corresponds to 1 millivolt.

    a.  1
    b.  3
    c.  5
    d.  10

62. EKG electrodes consist of a sticky outer margin and a _____ center to improve interface with the skin's surface.

    a.  saline
    b.  aluminum
    c.  gelled
    d.  glued

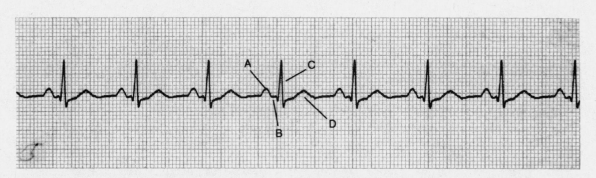

Match the EKG complex above with the appropriate type of wave or interval below:

d 63.  T wave                    C 65.  QRS

a 64.  P wave                    B 66.  PR interval

Review the tracings below and answer the questions that follow:

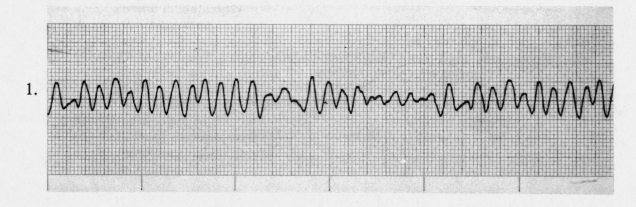

1.

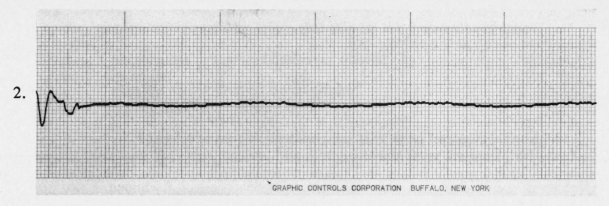

**2.**

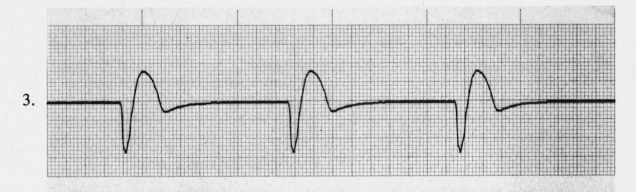

**3.**

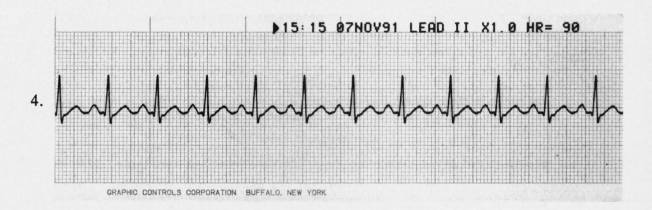

**4.**

15:15 07NOV91 LEAD II X1.0 HR= 90

67.    Which of the above rhythms require defibrillation?

    a.    1
    b.    2
    c.    3
    d.    4

68. Which two of the above rhythms may be found in electromechanical dissociation (EMD)?

    a. 1, 2
    b. 1, 3
    c. 2, 4
    d. 3, 4

69. The type of defibrillator that will identify the rhythm, charge and discharge automatically without any further direction from the operator is called:

    a. automatic
    b. semiautomatic
    c. manual
    d. controllable

70. Energy settings currently recommended by the American Heart Association (AHA) are ____ joules for the first defibrillation.

    a. 100
    b. 200
    c. 300
    d. 400

71. If ventricular fibrillation persists, AHA recommends_____ joules for the second defibrillation.

    a. 100-200
    b. 200-300
    c. 300-400
    d. 400-500

72. The recommended placement of paddles on the anterior chest wall is one positioned just below the right clavicle on the right sternal border and the other:

    a. just below the left clavicle
    b. directly over the mid-sternum
    c. just left of the left nipple, mid-axillary line
    d. just above the left nipple, mid-clavicular line

73. Which of the following is not considered an adequate approach to improving conduction across the skin?

    a. gels
    b. creams
    c. alcohol
    d. saline pads

74.    The transfer of electricity directly across the chest wall from one paddle to
       another via the conductive medium, sweat or other forms of moisture is
       called:

       a.    depolarization
       b.    bridging
       c.    resistance
       d.    repolarization

75.    To ensure firm contact between the paddle and the surface of the skin,
       approximately ____ pounds of muscular pressure is recommended?

       a.    5
       b.    10
       c.    15
       d.    25

76.    If the patient remains in ventricular fibrillation after the first defibrillation, it
       is generally recommended to:

       a.    perform CPR and transport
       b.    perform a precordial thump to stimulate the
             heart
       c.    defibrillate a second time at a higher setting
       d.    perform CPR for 10 minutes and defibrillate
             again

77.    If the patient converts to a organized rhythm (but does not have a pulse)
       following the defibrillation, the appropriate action would be to:

       a.    perform CPR and transport
       b.    perform a precordial thump to stimulate the heart
       c.    defibrillate a second time at a higher setting
       d.    perform CPR for 10 minutes and defibrillate
             again

Case Histories

| Case History #1 |
| --- |
| You respond to a call and find a 50 year old male who appears unresponsive. A bystander is performing one-rescuer CPR and tells you that the patient became unconscious 3 minutes ago, following a 15 minute episode of chest pain. |

78.    After performing one-rescuer CPR for 3 minutes, you note subcutaneous emphysema on the upper chest and neck.  What complication do you suspect?

    a.    airway or lung injury due to a fractured rib
    b.    cardiac contusion due to sternal compression
    c.    pericardial tamponade due to a fractured sternum
    d.    pulmonary embolus due to contusion from compressions

79.    Based on your impression of the underlying problem, your immediate actions should be to:

    a.    compress on the upper half of the sternum
    b.    stop CPR and transport immediately
    c.    ventilate and compress more forcefully
    d.    reevaluate your technique and continue CPR

---

### Case History #2

You respond to the home of a 65 year old patient who collapsed. On arrival, you find him alert and complaining of "squeezing" substernal chest pain for 20 minutes.  His skin is pale and cold; vital signs are blood pressure 110/70, respirations 24/min and pulse 75/min and regular. EKG shows:

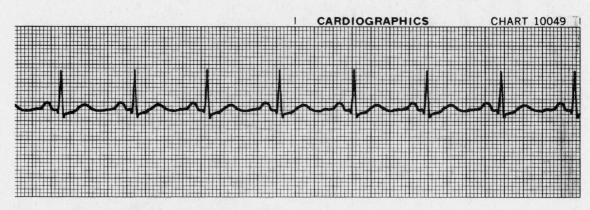

CARDIOGRAPHICS          CHART 10049

80.    Your prehospital impression is:

    a.    shock secondary to hemorrhage
    b.    myocardial infarction
    c.    angina pectoris
    d.    cerebral vascular accident

81. Your prehospital treatment would include:

    1. oxygen via nonrebreather mask
    2. precordial thump
    3. sitting position
    4. cardiac compressions

    a. 1, 2
    b. 1, 3
    c. 3, 4
    d. 2, 4

---

### Case History #2A

While enroute to the hospital, the patient becomes unconscious, pulseless and presents with this rhythm:

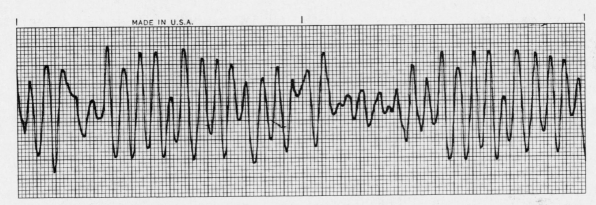

MADE IN U.S.A.

82. While your partner prepares the monitor-defibrillator, what immediate action should you take?

    a. administer oxygen via nonrebreather mask
    b. positive pressure ventilation
    c. administer a precordial thump
    d. insert an oropharyngeal airway

83. When the defibrillator is ready, what initial energy selection should be used (AHA standards)?

    a. 200 joules
    b. 300 joules
    c. 360 joules
    d. 400 joules

84.   You administer an immediate defibrillation, and sparks are ignited on the chest wall and you hear an explosive sound. You most likely used:

     a.   too high an energy level
     b.   too much conductive medium across the chest
     c.   too much pressure on the paddles
     d.   paddles that were too small

| Case History #2B |
| --- |
| You correct the problem and reevaluate the EKG and see the following: |

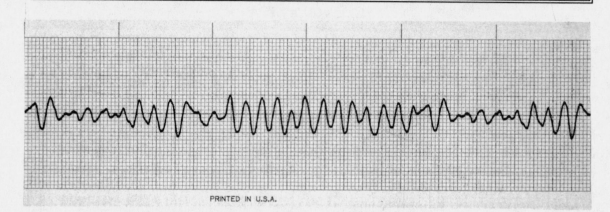

PRINTED IN U.S.A.

85.   The patient is still pulseless. Your next action is to:

     a.   administer a precordial thump
     b.   defibrillate at 200-300 joules
     c.   perform CPR and transport
     d.   defibrillate at 400 joules

| Case History #2C |
| --- |
| You initiate the above action and reevaluate the EKG, which shows the following: |

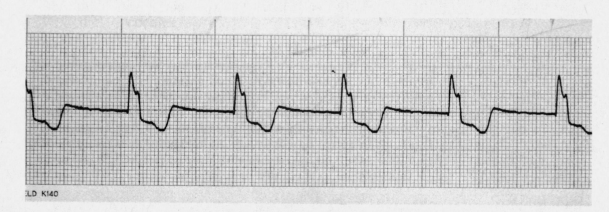

LD K140

86.    The patient is pulseless.  Your next action is to:

      a.     administer a precordial thump
      b.     defibrillate at 200-300 joules
      c.     perform CPR and transport
      d.     defibrillate at 400 joules

---

### Case History #3

You respond to a call and find a 55 year old male in cardiopulmonary arrest on the fifth floor of a building without an elevator.  You contact the dispatcher regarding the availability of a paramedic unit while your partner performs CPR. The dispatcher advises you that the paramedics are responding and will be at the scene within 4 minutes.  You attach the semiautomatic defibrillator to the patient, and the machine advises that defibrillation is needed.

---

87.    You defibrillate the patient and the machine advises you to defibrillate again. How many defibrillations should you provide prior to reevaluating the pulse?

      a.     1
      b.     2
      c.     3
      d.     4

88.    Given the situation, what would your actions be if the machine advised "no shock" and the patient were still pulseless?

      a.     do CPR and wait for the paramedic unit to arrive
      b.     transport immediately
      c.     continue defibrillating the patient
      d.     pronounce the patient dead

---

### Case History #4

A 58 year old male is found unresponsive and pulseless.  The ECG shows the following rhythm:

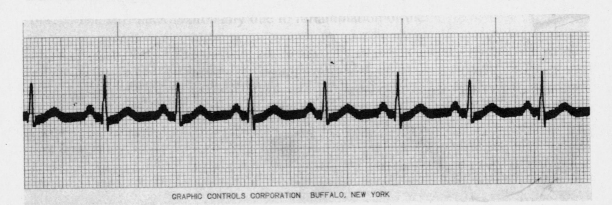

GRAPHIC CONTROLS CORPORATION  BUFFALO, NEW YORK

89.    Your appropriate action is to:

    a.    defibrillate
    b.    administer CPR and transport
    c.    transport without CPR
    d.    check the cables and patient

---

### Case History #5

A 57 year old female is found unresponsive and pulseless in the following rhythm:

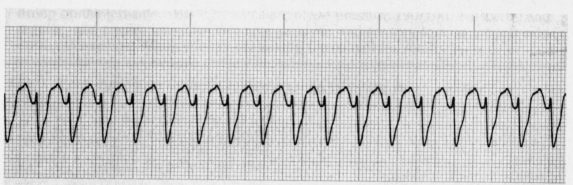

GRAPHIC C

90.    Which of the following statements is most true about this rhythm?

    a.    it always results in pulselessness
    b.    it never results in pulselessness
    c.    it may or may not result in pulselessness
    d.    it is a very stable rhythm

91.    Your appropriate action is to:

    a.    defibrillate
    b.    administer CPR and transport
    c.    transport without CPR
    d.    check the cables and patient for effective monitoring

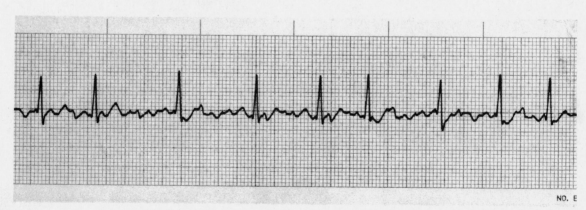

NO. E

92. How would you describe the above rhythm to a base station physician?

    a. regular
    b. regularly irregular
    c. irregularly irregular
    d. slightly irregular

93. A 55 year old male is found unresponsive <u>with</u> a pulse in the above rhythm. Your appropriate action is to:

    a. defibrillate
    b. administer CPR and transport
    c. transport without compressions
    d. administer a precordial thump

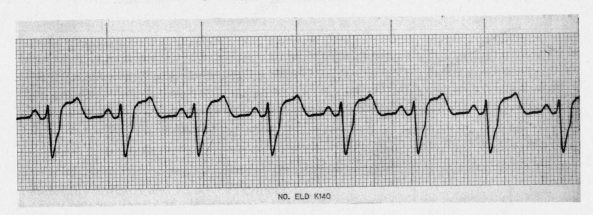

NO. ELD K140

94. A 58 year old male is found unresponsive and with a pulse in the above rhythm. Your appropriate action is to:

    a. defibrillate
    b. administer CPR and transport
    c. transport without CPR
    d. check the cables and patient for effective monitoring technique

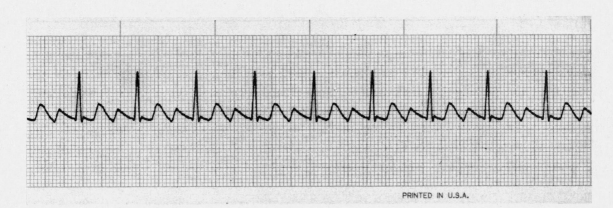

PRINTED IN U.S.A.

95.     A 66 year old female is found unresponsive with a pulse in the above rhythm. Your appropriate action is to:

    a.     defibrillate
    b.     administer CPR and transport
    c.     transport without CPR
    d.     check the cables and patient for effective monitoring technique

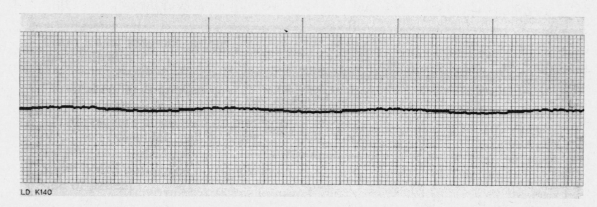

LD K140

96.     A 47 year old male is found in the above rhythm on a manual defibrillator. What action should you take to see if defibrillation may be necessary?

    a.     change the selected lead
    b.     reapply the electrodes
    c.     shake the patient cable
    d.     change the patient cable

Skill Performance Sheet

**Adult One-Rescuer CPR**

Student Name_____          Date_____

| Performance Standard | Performed | Failed |
|---|---|---|
| Establish unresponsiveness, open airway with appropriate maneuver (head tilt-chin lift or jaw thrust) | | |
| Assess breathing (look, listen and feel) | | |
| Seal mouth around the patient's mouth and pinch nose | | |
| Give two smooth breaths while observing chest rise (1-1.5 seconds per breath) | | |
| Take mouth away between breaths | | |
| Check carotid pulse (pulse is absent) | | |
| If no pulse, locate correct hand position | | |
| Maintain vertical position and provide 15 compressions (80-100/min) | | |
| Provide two ventilations | | |
| After four cycles of 15:2, give two ventilations and check a pulse | | |
| If no pulse, continue 15:2 cycle | | |

Comments_____

_____

_____

_____

Instructor _____          Circle One:   Pass   Fail

Skill Performance Sheet

**Adult Two-Rescuer CPR**

Student Name_____          Date_____

| Performance Standard | Performed | Failed |
|---|---|---|
| **RESCUER #1** | | |
| Open airway with appropriate maneuver (head tilt-chin lift or jaw thrust) | | |
| Assess breathing (look, listen and feel) | | |
| Seal mouth around the patient's mouth and pinch nose | | |
| Give two smooth breaths while observing chest rise (1-1.5 seconds per breath) | | |
| Take mouth away between breaths | | |
| Check carotid pulse (pulse is absent) | | |
| **RESCUER #2** | | |
| If no pulse, locate correct hand position | | |
| Maintain vertical position and provide five compressions (80-100/min) | | |
| Rescuer #1 provide one ventilation | | |
| After four cycles of 5:1, check a pulse | | |
| If no pulse, continue 5:1 cycle | | |

Comments_____

_____

Instructor _____          Circle One:   Pass   Fail

*CPR and Defibrillation*

Skill Performance Sheet

**Child One-Rescuer CPR**

Student Name_____          Date_____

| Performance Standard | Performed | Failed |
|---|---|---|
| Open airway with appropriate maneuver (head tilt-chin lift or jaw thrust) | | |
| Assess breathing (look, listen and feel) | | |
| Seal mouth around the patient's mouth and pinch nose | | |
| Give two smooth breaths while observing chest rise (1-1.5 seconds per breath) | | |
| Take mouth away between breaths | | |
| Check carotid pulse (pulse is absent) | | |
| If no pulse, locate correct hand position | | |
| Maintain vertical position and provide five compressions (80-100/min) while continuing to maintain head tilt | | |
| Provide one ventilation | | |
| After ten cycles of 5:1, give two ventilations and check a pulse | | |
| If no pulse, continue 5:1 cycle | | |

Comments_____

_____

_____

Instructor _____          Circle One:   Pass   Fail

Skill Performance Sheet

**Infant One-Rescuer CPR**

Student Name_____          Date_____

| Performance Standard | Performed | Failed |
|---|---|---|
| Open airway with appropriate maneuver (head tilt-chin lift or jaw thrust) | | |
| Assess breathing (look, listen and feel) | | |
| Seal mouth around the patient's mouth and nose | | |
| Give two smooth breaths while observing chest rise (1-1.5 seconds per breath) | | |
| Take mouth away between breaths | | |
| Check brachial pulse (pulse is absent) | | |
| Locate correct finger position (one finger below nipple line) | | |
| Maintain head tilt | | |
| Provide compressions at a rate of 100/min (1/2 to 1 inch) | | |
| Perform ten cycles at 5:1 ratio | | |
| Check pulse | | |
| If no pulse, continue CPR | | |

Comments_____

_____

_____

Instructor _____          Circle One:   Pass   Fail

Skill Performance Sheet

## Defibrillation - Manual Defibrillator

Student Name_____          Date_____

| Performance Standard | Performed | Failed |
|---|---|---|
| Check for pulselessness | | |
| If witnessed arrest, perform precordial thump | | |
| If pulseless, EMT #1 perform CPR | | |
| EMT #2: attaches electrodes and leads | | |
| Turn on recorder and medical control device | | |
| Assess rhythm | | |
| If ventricular fibrillation or ventricular tachycardia, proceed: | | |
| Apply gel or other conductive medium to paddles | | |
| Charge paddles to 200 joules | | |
| Properly place paddles and apply 25 pounds of muscular pressure | | |
| Announce "all clear" and confirm that no person is in contact with the patient | | |
| Press the discharge buttons and defibrillate | | |
| Reevaluate pulse and rhythm | | |
| If still in ventricular fibrillation or ventricular tachycardia, repeat defibrillation process at 200-300 joules. | | |

CONTINUED ON NEXT PAGE

Skill Performance Sheet

**Defibrillation - Manual Defibrillator (continued)**

| Performance Standard | Performed | Failed |
|---|---|---|
| Reevaluate pulse and rhythm | | |
| If still in ventricular fibrillation or ventricular tachycardia, repeat defibrillation process at 360-400 joules | | |
| Reevaluate pulse and rhythm | | |
| Continue according to local protocol | | |

Comments_____

_____

_____

_____

Instructor _____     Circle One:   Pass   Fail

Skill Performance Sheet

## Defibrillation - Semiautomatic Defibrillator

Student Name_____          Date_____

| Performance Standard | Performed | Failed |
|---|---|---|
| Check pulselessness | | |
| If witnessed arrest, perform precordial thump | | |
| If pulseless, EMT #1 perform CPR | | |
| EMT #2 attaches electrodes and leads | | |
| Turn on device | | |
| Push analyze and stand clear of patient | | |
| If ventricular fibrillation or ventricular tachycardia, the machine will advise defibrillation | | |
| Machine will either charge or advise operator to charge (200 joules) | | |
| Announce "all clear" and confirm that no person is in contact with the patient | | |
| Press the discharge buttons | | |
| Push analyze and stand clear of patient | | |
| If ventricular fibrillation or ventricular tachycardia, the machine will advise defibrillation | | |
| Machine will either charge or advise operator to charge (300 joules) | | |

CONTINUED ON NEXT PAGE

Skill Performance Sheet

**Defibrillation - Semiautomatic Defibrillator (continued)**

| Performance Standard | Performed | Failed |
|---|---|---|
| Announce "all clear" and confirm that no person is in contact with the patient | | |
| Press the discharge buttons | | |
| Push analyze and stand clear of patient | | |
| If ventricular fibrillation or ventricular tachycardia, the machine will advise defibrillation | | |
| Machine will either charge or advise operator to charge (360 joules) | | |
| Announce "all clear" and confirm that no person is in contact with the patient | | |
| Press the discharge buttons | | |
| Reevaluate pulse and rhythm | | |
| If pulseless, perform CPR for 1 minute | | |
| If still in ventricular fibrillation or ventricular tachycardia, repeat process of three stacked shocks at 360 joules. | | |
| Continue process according to local protocol | | |

Comments_____

_____

_____

Instructor _____     Circle One:   Pass   Fail

# CENTRAL NERVOUS SYSTEM EMERGENCIES

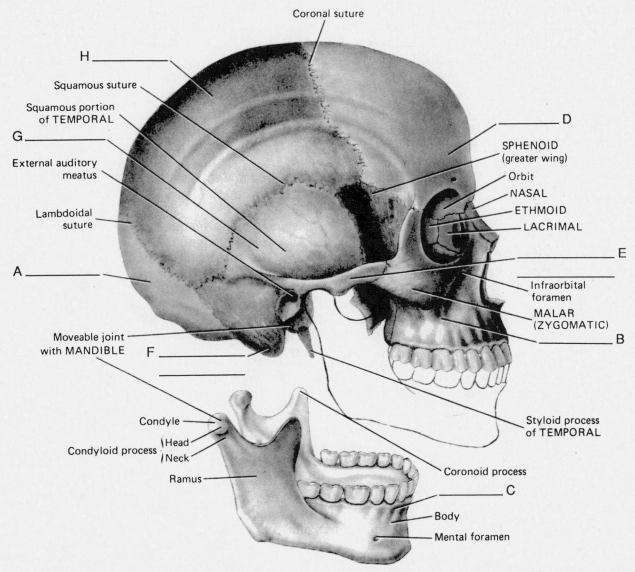

Coronal suture

H

Squamous suture

Squamous portion
of TEMPORAL

G

External auditory
meatus

Lambdoidal
suture

A

D

SPHENOID
(greater wing)

Orbit
NASAL
ETHMOID
LACRIMAL

E

Infraorbital
foramen

MALAR
(ZYGOMATIC)

B

Moveable joint
with MANDIBLE

F

Condyle
Condyloid process — Head
Neck
Ramus

Coronoid process

Styloid process
of TEMPORAL

C

Body

Mental foramen

(Solomon EP, Phillips GA: Understanding Human Anatomy and Physiology. Philadelphia, WB Saunders, 1987, p81)

Match the bones on the drawing above to the terms below.

*a* 1. occipital

*6* 2. temporal

*H* 3. parietal

*C* 4. mandible

*D* 5. frontal

*F* 6. mastoid process

*E* 7. zygomatic process

*B* 8. maxilla

9.  The nervous system is structurally divided into two main divisions -- the central nervous system and the _____ nervous system.

    a.  peripheral
    b.  ganglionic
    c.  proximal
    d.  core

10. The central nervous system is made up of the brain, the brainstem and the:

    a.  afferent nerves
    b.  peripheral nerves
    c.  dermatomes
    d.  spinal cord

11. The nervous system can also be divided by function, creating the voluntary and _____ divisions.

    a.  paravoluntary
    b.  autonomic
    c.  reflex
    d.  ganglionic

12. Willful activities such as running to catch a train, reaching for an object or buttoning a shirt are examples of functions mediated through the _____ division of the nervous system.

    a.  autonomic
    b.  reflex
    c.  spinal
    d.  voluntary

13. The control of the heart, the glands and smooth muscles within organs such as the digestive tract is mediated through the _____ division of the nervous system.

    a.  autonomic
    b.  reflex
    c.  spinal
    d.  voluntary

14. There are two main divisions of the autonomic nervous system -- the parasympathetic and the:

    a.  paraspinal
    b.  parasympathomimetic
    c.  sympathetic
    d.  sympathomimetic

15. Which of the following is mediated through the parasympathetic nervous system?

    a. sweating
    b. constriction of pupils
    c. increasing the heart rate
    d. vasoconstriction

16. If complete cessation of oxygen delivery occurs, as in cardiac arrest, the patient will become unconscious in about:

    a. 5 seconds
    b. 1 minute
    c. 4-6 minutes
    d. 10 minutes

17. Approximately how long will it take for irreversible brain damage to occur when the brain is totally deprived of oxygen?

    a. 5-10 seconds
    b. 1-2 minutes
    c. 2-3 minutes
    d. 4-6 minutes

18. The most sensitive indicator of inadequate oxygenation of the brain is:

    a. alteration of mental status
    b. motor function
    c. sensory function
    d. heart rate

Match the regions of the skull in column B with their related bones in column A. You can use the column B selections more than once.

| Column A | | Column B | |
|---|---|---|---|
| B 19. | mandible | a. | cranium |
| A 20. | parietal | b. | face |
| B 21. | maxilla | | |
| A 22. | temporal | | |
| A 23. | occipital | | |

24.     The brainstem exits the lower skull through an opening called the:

       a.      foramen arteriosum
       b.     foramen magnum
       c.      foramen ovale
       d.      foramen minor

25.     The space <u>within</u> the adult cranium has about a _____ capacity.

       a.      0.5 liter
       b.     1.0 liter
       c.      2.0 liter
       d.      3.0 liter

26.     If the pressure within the cranium becomes severe, the brain may be forced down through the opening in the base of the skull. This dire emergency is called:

       a.      displacement
       b.     herniation
       c.      pressure syndrome
       d.      compression syndrome

Match the number of vertebrae in column B with the type of vertebrae in column A.

| Column A | | Column B | |
| --- | --- | --- | --- |
| E 27. | cervical | a. | 5 (mobile) |
| A 28. | lumbar | b. | 4 (fused) |
| B 29. | coccyx | c. | 12 |
| D 30. | sacral | d. | 5 (fused) |
| C 31. | thoracic | e. | 7 |

32.     Most vertebrae are held together by ligaments and separated by _____ that serve as cushions.

       a.      discs
       b.     nerves
       c.      bone
       d.      tendons

33.    The three layered membranous coverings of the brain and spinal cord that serve to protect the central nervous system are called the:

a.    pleura
b.    periosteum
c.    myelin sheath
d.    meninges

Match the description in column B to the appropriate membranous layer in column A.

| Column A | Column B |
| --- | --- |
| C 34.    pia mater | a.    tough, leathery outer layer |
| B 35.    arachnoid | b.    middle layer |
| A 36.    dura mater | c.    inner layer |

37.    The largest and most superior portion of the brain is called the:

a.    cerebrum
b.    brainstem
c.    cerebellum
d.    diencephalon

38.    The lower part of the brain that is made up of bundles and tracts of nerves traveling down to the spinal cord and has distinct nerve cell centers of its own is called the:

a.    cerebrum
b.    brainstem
c.    cerebellum
d.    diencephalon

39.    The posterior outpocketing of the brain that is primarily concerned with coordination of movement and balance is called the:

a.    cerebrum
b.    brainstem
c.    cerebellum
d.    diencephalon

Match the type of action mediated by the central nervous system in column B to the category in column A.

Column A                                         Column B

A   40.    automatic              a.    breathing, heart rate, etc.

B   41.    reflex                 b.    withdrawal from hot candle

C   42.    conscious              c.    lifting a box

D   43.    Most of the blood supply to the brain (80%) is provided through the
           _____ arteries.

           a.    vertebral
           b.    subleasing
           c.    middle meningeal
           d.    carotid

Match the functions in column B with the appropriate area of the brain in column A.

Column A                                         Column B

B   44.    frontal lobe           a.    vision

D   45.    parietal lobe          b.    intellect -- motor
                                       function

A   46.    occipital lobe
                           c.    respiratory function

C   47.    brain stem
                           d.    sensory function

E   48.    temporal lobe
                           e.    hearing, smell

49.    Injuries that cause disruption of <u>specific</u> sections of brain tissue or nerves (i.e., gunshot wounds) and result in loss of specific functions are called _____ injuries.

           a.    metabolic
           b.    secondary
           c.    structural
           d.    contained

50.    Problems that affect all of the brain cells equally, such as hypoxia, low blood sugar, shock and poisoning, are called _____ injuries.

           a.    metabolic
           b.    secondary
           c.    structural
           d.    contained

51.    Hypoxia, hypotension, hypoglycemia, infections and increased intracranial pressure are all examples of _____ brain injuries.

    a.    secondary
    b.    primary
    c.    modifying
    d.    complicating

52.    Injuries that occur on the <u>opposite</u> side of the brain from the site of the blow (due to the dynamic movement of the brain following initial impact) are called _____ injuries.

    a.    compression
    b.    deceleration
    c.    contrecoup
    d.    ipsilateral contusion

Match the description in column B to the type of skull fracture in column A.

| Column A | | Column B | |
| --- | --- | --- | --- |
| C 53. | linear | a. | a crack in the floor of the skull |
| A 54. | basilar | | |
| D 55. | comminuted | b. | bone fragments that are pressed downward toward the brain |
| B 56. | depressed | | |
| | | c. | a line of non-union along the cranium |
| | | d. | multiple cracks radiating outward from the point of impact |

57.    Cerebrospinal fluid leaking from the ear should be treated by:

    a.    packing the ear to contain fluid
    b.    attaching a loose dressing over the ear
    c.    doing nothing
    d.    placing the patient on the affected side

58.    Raccoon eyes, Battle's sign and cerebrospinal fluid leakage from the nose or ear are all signs of:

    a.    brain laceration
    b.    epidural hematoma
    c.    basilar skull fracture
    d.    increased intracranial pressure

59. A transient loss of consciousness or neurological function due to a blow to the brain is called a:

    a. contusion
    b. concussion
    c. compression
    d. contortion

60. Headaches, nausea and vomiting (sometimes projectile) are common signs of _____ in the conscious head trauma patient.

    a. skull fracture
    b. brain contusion
    c. increased intracranial pressure
    d. infection

61. Which of the following vital sign presentations may signify an increase in intracranial pressure?

    a. decreased pulse rate, increased blood pressure
    b. increased pulse rate, decreased blood pressure
    c. decreased pulse rate, decreased blood pressure
    d. increased pulse rate, increased blood pressure

62. Epidural hematomas are caused by _____ bleeding.

    a. arterial
    b. capillary
    c. venous
    d. venule

63. Subdural hematomas are caused by _____ bleeding.

    a. arterial
    b. capillary
    c. venous
    d. venule

64. A loss of consciousness, followed by a lucid interval, followed by a subsequent loss of consciousness suggests:

    a. a brain contusion
    b. an expanding hematoma
    c. a concussion
    d. a fractured skull

65.     A traumatic eye problem that may affect both the size of the pupil and its
        ability to react to light is called:

        a.      glaucoma
        b.      central retinal artery occlusion
        c.      traumatic iritis
        d.      sclera hematoma

66.     The manual airway maneuver of choice for the head injured patient is:

        a.      head tilt-chin lift
        b.      head tilt-neck lift
        c.      jaw thrust without head tilt (modified)
        d.      triple airway maneuver

67.     Increased levels of carbon dioxide causes _____ of cerebral vessels.

        a.      constriction
        b.      dilation
        c.      spasm
        d.      obstruction

68.     The Glasgow coma scale for a patient who has no verbalizations, does not
        open his eyes and who is decorticate (has abnormal flexion) to painful stimuli
        is:

        a.      4
        b.      5
        c.      7
        d.      9

69.     The first priority in the management of a patient with a severe head trauma
        is:

        a.      performing a neurological exam
        b.      establishing an airway and adequate ventilation
        c.      applying a cervical collar
        d.      controlling bleeding from the scalp

Match the anatomic sensory area (dermatome) in column B with the appropriate
spinal nerve level in column A

| Column A | | Column B | |
|---|---|---|---|
| B 70. | thoracic 4 (T-4) | a. | groin |
| C 71. | cervical 4 (C-4) | b. | nipple |
| A 72. | lumbar 1 (L-1) | c. | above clavicle |
| D 73. | thoracic 10 (T-10) | d. | umbilicus |

74. When the spinal cord is injured at a <u>low cervical level (C-7) or a high thoracic level (T-1)</u>, the respiratory function is most likely to be:

    a. respiratory arrest
    b. intercostal breathing only
    c. diaphragmatic breathing only
    d. normal respiration

75. When the spinal cord is injured at a <u>high cervical level (C-2)</u>, the respiratory function is most likely to be:

    a. respiratory arrest
    b. intercostal breathing only
    c. diaphragmatic breathing only
    d. normal respiration

76. When a patient develops neurogenic shock secondary to spinal injuries, the pulse rate is most likely to be:

    a. slow (below 60)
    b. normal range (60-80)
    c. fast (above 100)
    d. very fast (above 150)

77. The vessels of a patient in neurogenic shock are most likely to be:

    a. constricted
    b. dilated
    c. normal
    d. collapsed

78. The loss of sympathetic tone of a patient in neurogenic shock may result in a penile erection. This event is commonly called:

    a. neuroerection
    b. priaprism
    c. sympathetic erection
    d. penile dilation

79. The most common cause of spinal cord injury is:

    a. motor vehicle accidents
    b. falls
    c. sports-related accidents
    d. diving accidents

80.    The most common sites of vertebral injury occur where vertebrae that allow motion meet:

    a.    the rib cage
    b.    vertebrae that are fixed
    c.    other mobile vertebrae
    d.    intervertebral discs

Match the mechanisms of injury in column B to the appropriate type of spinal injury force in column A.

| Column A | | Column B |
| --- | --- | --- |
| *C* 81. compression | a. | face striking the windshield in a frontend collision |
| *B* 82. flexion | | |
| | b. | occipital region striking the bottom of a pool during a dive |
| *A* 83. extension | | |
| | c. | the top portion of the skull striking the bottom of a pool during a dive |

84.    The term used to describe a <u>hyperextension</u> injury resulting from a rearend collision is:

    a.    contrecoup
    b.    whiplash
    c.    posterior extension
    d.    subluxation

85.    When immobilizing a spinal injury victim you <u>should not</u> return the neck to the neutral position if:

    a.    the neck is flexed
    b.    resistance is encountered
    c.    the neck is extended
    d.    contusions are noted on the neck

Match the situation in column B to the approach to immobilization in column A.

| Column A | | Column B |
| --- | --- | --- |
| *C* 86. short board | a. | unstable driver of a car |
| *B* 87. long board | b. | pedestrian struck by |
| *A* 88. rapid extrication | c. | stable driver of a car |

Match the definition in column B to the term in column A.

| Column A | | Column B |
| --- | --- | --- |

B 89.   lethargy

    a.    a state of lessened responsiveness where patient can be aroused but more stimuli is required

A 90.   stupor

    b.    sluggishness or sleepiness

C 91.  coma

    c.    a lack of responsiveness to the environment

92.   A blockage or disruption of blood flow in an artery feeding the brain best defines:

    a.    epidural hematoma
    b.    encephalitis
    c.    cerebral vascular accident
    d.    aneurysm

93.   The most common cause of a CVA is:

    a.    hemorrhage
    b.    thrombus
    c.    embolus
    d.    spasm

94.   A type of stroke that results from a traveling blood clot's becoming lodged in a particular area of the brain's blood supply is called a(n) _____ stroke.

    a.    hemorrhagic
    b.    thrombotic
    c.    embolotic
    d.    ischemic

95.   The type of stroke that has the highest death rate is a(n) _____ stroke.

    a.    hemorrhagic
    b.    thrombotic
    c.    embolotic
    d.    ischemic

96.   A temporary loss of brain function secondary to diminished blood supply to part of the brain that resolves within 12 hours of onset best defines:

    a.    transient ischemic attack (TIA)
    b.    CVA
    c.    cerebral insufficiency
    d.    cerebral obstruction

97.   Neck stiffness is most commonly related to which of the following neurological problems?

      a.   seizures
      b.   thrombotic stroke
      c.   subarachnoid hemorrhage
      d.   embolotic stroke

98.   The most common motor finding in the extremities following a stroke is:

      a.   paraplegia
      b.   hemiplegia
      c.   quadraplegia
      d.   normal findings

99.   A stroke in the left cerebral hemisphere is likely to result in:

      a.   right-sided arm weakness
      b.   left-sided arm weakness
      c.   bilateral arm weakness
      d.   no arm weakness

100.  A temporary alteration in behavior due to abnormal electrical activity in the brain best defines:

      a.   a stroke
      b.   a subarachnoid hemorrhage
      c.   meningitis
      d.   a seizure

101.  Which of the following drugs are commonly used in the treatment of epilepsy?

      a.   xylocaine and atropine
      b.   epinephrine and isoproterenol
      c.   dextrose and reserpine
      d.   phenobarbital and dilantin

Match the descriptions in column B with the phases of a seizure in column A.

| Column A | | Column B | |
|---|---|---|---|
| C 102. | postictal | a. | sustained contraction of all voluntary muscles |
| B 103. | clonic | b. | intermittent contractions and relaxations of the skeletal muscles |
| A 104. | tonic | c. | sleepy depressed level of consciousness and confusion |

105. Strange smells, visual or auditory sensations, or motor events that may herald the onset of a seizure are commonly referred to as:

    a. preconvulsion phenomena
    b. an aura
    c. status epilepticus
    d. petite mal event

106. A seizure that affects only a portion of the body is called a _____ seizure.

    a. manic
    b. focal
    c. petite mal
    d. febrile

107. A rapid succession of epileptic attacks without an intervening period of consciousness is called:

    a. status epilepticus
    b. psychomotor convulsion
    c. epilepsy
    d. petite mal epilepsy

108. Febrile convulsions most commonly occur in:

    a. pregnant women
    b. alcoholics
    c. children
    d. athletes

109. Brief lapses of attention and awareness lasting 10-20 seconds that are more common in childhood but sometimes persist into adult life are called:

    a. status epilepticus
    b. grand mal epilepsy
    c. petite mal epilepsy
    d. focal seizures

110. Which of the following signs would provide the "green light" for insertion of an oropharyngeal airway during the postictal phase of a seizure?

    a. active swallowing reflex
    b. absent gag reflex
    c. lethargic mental state
    d. movement of the larynx

111. An infection of the <u>brain coverings</u> that may be life threatening is called:

    a. encephalitis
    b. neuritis
    c. duraitis
    d. meningitis

112. A change in mental status, severe headache, stiff neck, photophobia (bright light irritates the eyes), nausea, loss of appetite and fever are most likely the result of:

    a. stroke
    b. encephalitis
    c. meningitis
    d. subarachnoid hemorrhage

113. The most treatable and also most common hazard faced by patients with altered mental function is:

    a. respiratory arrest
    b. airway compromise
    c. bleeding
    d. increased intracranial pressure

114. Patients with an altered mental status and cyanosis or evidence of respiratory distress should receive oxygen via a:

    a. nasal cannula
    b. partial rebreather mask
    c. simple face mask
    d. nonrebreather mask

115. In systems with prehospital ALS, patients with altered mental states are routinely treated with:

    a. dilantin
    b. dextrose
    c. epinephrine
    d. phenobarbital

## Case Histories

| Case History #1 |
| --- |
| A 25 year old unconscious male was involved in a motor vehicle accident. Bystanders state that he was initially unconscious, became conscious 3 minutes after the accident and lapsed into unconsciousness again about 5 minutes ago. He is unresponsive to pain. Physical assessment reveals left pupil dilated and nonreactive; blood pressure 200/110, pulse 42 and bounding, and respirations irregular at an approximate rate of 8/min. He has a contusion and crepitus in the temporal region of the skull. |

116. What do you suspect is the major underlying problem?

    a.     brain contusion
    b.     epidural hematoma
    c.     concussion
    d.     subdural hematoma

117. The characteristic change in blood pressure and pulse rate is known as:

    a.     Homan's signs
    b.     Battle's signs
    c.     Cushing's reflex
    d.     the raccoon reflex

118. What is the likely cause of the change in vital signs?

    a.     increased intracranial pressure
    b.     direct injury to the brain
    c.     the age of the patient
    d.     a history of hypertension

119. The respiratory pattern best describes _____ breathing.

    a.     ataxic
    b.     Biot's
    c.     Cheyenne-Stokes
    d.     central neurogenic hyperventilation

120. Which of the following best describes the sequential treatment of this patient?

    a.     rapid extrication, positive pressure ventilation (25/min), long spine board, transport
    b.     short spine board, oxygen via nonrebreather mask, long spine board, transport
    c.     oxygen nonrebreather mask, rapid extrication, long spine board, transport
    d.     positive pressure ventilation, PSAG, short spine board, transport

---

### Case History #2

A 14 year old falls approximately 7 feet from a swing and strikes his left forehead on a soft rubber mat, causing him to become unconscious. After 30 seconds, he awakes and says he feels "all right." You find the youngster alert and breathing with his abdominal muscles only. Vital signs are pulse 68 and regular, and blood pressure 76/60. He cannot move his arms and legs and has sensation above the clavicle but none at nipple line. You also note priaprism.

---

121. Based on the presenting signs you suspect spinal injury at the level of the:

    a. high thoracic or low cervical spine
    b. low thoracic or high lumbar spine
    c. high cervical spine
    d. low lumbar or high sacral spine

122. Based on the vital signs, what complication do you suspect?

    a. increased intracranial pressure
    b. neurogenic (spinal) shock
    c. obstructive shock
    d. epidural hematoma

123. The vital signs, priaprism and loss of the sweat mechanism below the clavicles are a result of:

    a. increased parasympathetic activity
    b. increased sympathetic activity
    c. decreased parasympathetic activity
    d. decreased sympathetic activity

124. His respiratory status is due to a loss of _____ function.

    a. diaphragm
    b. intercostal muscle
    c. abdominal muscle
    d. neck muscle

125. The initial loss of consciousness is probably due to a:

    a. contusion
    b. laceration
    c. concussion
    d. epidural bleeding

126. Treatment of this patient should include spinal immobilization,

    a.  oxygen via nonrebreather mask
    b.  oxygen via nasal cannula
    c.  oxygen via Venturi mask
    d.  no oxygen

---

### Case History #3

A 40 year old man was in a frontend auto collision and lost consciousness. When the ambulance arrived, the patient refused medical evaluation and treatment. A week later, the man became unconscious while watching TV at home. Upon your arrival on the scene, the patient is unresponsive to painful stimuli. His vital signs are blood pressure 150/100, respirations 36/min and very deep and pulse 80. His left pupil is fixed and dilated and his right is midpositional and normally reactive.

---

127. Based on the history and presenting signs, what do you think is the primary problem?

    a.  cerebral contusion
    b.  stroke
    c.  subdural hematoma
    d.  subarachnoid hemorrhage

128. The bleeding within the skull is most likely:

    a.  arterial
    b.  capillary
    c.  venous
    d.  arteriole

129. The initial loss of consciousness following the accident was probably due to a:

    a.  concussion
    b.  contusion
    c.  laceration
    d.  abrasion

130. The respiratory pattern best describes:

    a.  Cheyenne-Stokes breathing
    b.  ataxic ventilation
    c.  Biot's breathing
    d.  central neurogenic hyperventilation

131.  Based on the ventilatory status, what approach would you use to deliver oxygen?

      a.   nasal cannula
      b.   nonrebreather mask
      c.   bag-valve-mask
      d.   simple face mask

---

### Case History #4

You find a 60 year old woman alert and oriented on a couch in her apartment. Her daughter advises you that this morning she developed weakness on the left side of her body and difficulty speaking that lasted for about 1 hour. Upon physical assessment you note normal motor and sensory function. Her vital signs are blood pressure 170/105, respirations 17/min and regular, and pulse 80/min. The patient has a past medical history of high blood pressure, diabetes, high blood cholesterol and bronchitis.

---

132.  Based on the history and physical assessment, the most likely cause of her problem is:

      a.   stroke
      b.   transient ischemic attack
      c.   subarachnoid hemorrhage
      d.   subdural hematoma

133.  Her problem is most likely related to:

      a.   a thrombus in her cerebral artery
      b.   a hemorrhage in her brain
      c.   her current blood pressure
      d.   her position at the time of the event

134.  Which of the elements of the past medical history is <u>not</u> a risk factor of her condition?

      a.   high blood pressure
      b    diabetes
      c.   high blood cholesterol
      d.   bronchitis

135.  Given the circumstances, you would advise her to:

      a.   come to the hospital for evaluation
      b.   not seek medical attention
      c.   call her doctor when she gets a chance
      d.   observe for reoccurrence and call again

---

### Case History #5

You find a 25 year old man unresponsive to painful stimuli at work. His co-workers advise you that he had what appeared to be a convulsion that lasted for 3 minutes with his entire body contracting and relaxing intermittently 5 minutes prior to your arrival. His vital signs are blood pressure 140/95, respirations 24/min and deep, and pulse 94 and regular. The co-workers state that he had no known significant medical history. The police search the patient and find medications including phenobarbital and dilantin.

---

136. Based on the age of the patient and the description of the event, what do you suspect?

    a.    petite mal seizure
    b.    grand mal seizure
    c.    focal seizure
    d.    febrile seizure

137. What phase of the seizure is the patient in at this time?

    a.    tonic
    b.    clonic
    c.    aura
    d.    posticthal

138. What can you search for that may provide further evidence to confirm your impression?

    a.    incontinence and tongue biting
    b.    dilated pupils and paralysis on one side
    c.    stiff neck and fever
    d.    decorticate posturing and sensory deficits

139. The medications are:

    a.    antiemetics
    b.    anticonvulsants
    c.    antibiotics
    d.    antidepressants

---

### Case History #5A

While you are evaluating the patient, he becomes extremely stiff for about 30 seconds and then begins to alternately contract and relax his muscles in his extremities and neck. He appears to stop breathing during the first 30 seconds but is moving some air during this phase of the seizure.

---

140.    Based on this event, you suspect:

      a.     status epilepticus
      b.     recurrent febrile convulsions
      c.     posticthal contractions
      d.     a focal seizure

141.    The first phase of this event, in which the patient became extremely stiff and appeared to stop breathing for 30 seconds, best describes the _____ phase of a seizure.

      a.     tonic
      b.     clonic
      c.     posticthal
      d.     aura

142.    What is your greatest concern about this patient?

      a.     he may rupture a brain vessel
      b.     his ability to ventilate adequately
      c.     injury to his extremities
      d.     he may develop a pneumothorax due to his straining

---

### Case History #6

You find an 8 year old febrile girl responsive to painful but not verbal stimuli. The parents advise you that she has been sick for two days with a fever, headache, photophobia (irritation to light), nausea, loss of appetite and a stiff neck. Her vital signs are blood pressure 130/70, pulse 100 and regular, and respirations 24. She is hot to the touch, and her neck is stiff and painful when flexion is attempted.

---

143.    Based on the history and physical assessment, you suspect:

      a.     subarachnoid hemorrhage
      b.     epilepsy
      c.     meningitis
      d.     subdural hematoma

144.    The stiff neck is probably due to inflammation of the:

      a.     brain tissues
      b.     CNS coverings
      c.     inner lining of the skull
      d.     spinal cord

145. Caution should be exercised in the management of this patient since her condition may:

  a. cause immediate cardiac arrest
  b. be communicable
  c. lead to a stroke
  d. cause intracerebral bleeding

---

### Case History #7

You find a 78 year old male responsive to verbal stimuli with paralysis on the left side of his body. His wife advises you that she found him like this when she woke him this morning. He is able to speak but slurs his words and has a facial droop on the left side. His vital signs are blood pressure 190/100, pulse 100 and regular, and respirations 24. You note paralysis and sensory loss on the left side during the exam. While you are examining the patient he vomits.

---

146. Your immediate action in response to the vomiting is:

  a. turn the patient on his side
  b. turn the patient facedown
  c. leave the patient supine
  d. stand the patient upright

147. Based on the history and physical assessment, you suspect:

  a. transient ischemic attack
  b. CVA (cerebrovascular accident)
  c. encephalitis
  d. meningitis

148. Considering this patient's mental status, the best method for continuous management of this patient's airway is:

  a. oropharyngeal airway insertion
  b. esophageal airway
  c. left lateral recumbent positioning
  d. endotracheal intubation

Skill Performance Sheet

**Helmet Removal**

Student Name_____       Date_____

| Performance Standard | Performed | Failed |
|---|---|---|
| **EMT #1** | | |
| Maintains in-line immobilization with helmet | | |
| **EMT #2** | | |
| Cuts or removes chin strap | | |
| Supports occipital area with arm on ground | | |
| Supports mandible along bony margin | | |
| **EMT #1** | | |
| Laterally spreads and removes helmet (may rotate slightly to clear nose) | | |
| Takes over in-line immobilization (may place towel under occipital area) | | |

Comments_____

_____

_____

_____

Instructor _____       Circle One:   Pass   Fail

## Skill Performance Sheet

## **Log Roll Procedure**

Student Name_____          Date_____

| Performance Standard | Performed | Failed |
|---|---|---|
| Team leader assumes in-line immobilization | | |
| Cervical collar is applied | | |
| Three rescuers positioned on one side of patient (shoulder, pelvis, legs) | | |
| Spine board positioned on opposite side of patient | | |
| On command from team leader, patient is rolled toward three rescuers | | |
| Board is slid under patient | | |
| On command from team leader, patient is rolled onto board | | |
| Patient is adjusted on board | | |
| Body then head is securely attached to spine board | | |

Comments_____

_____

_____

_____

Instructor _____          Circle One:  Pass  Fail

# Chapter 8

## ABDOMINAL EMERGENCIES

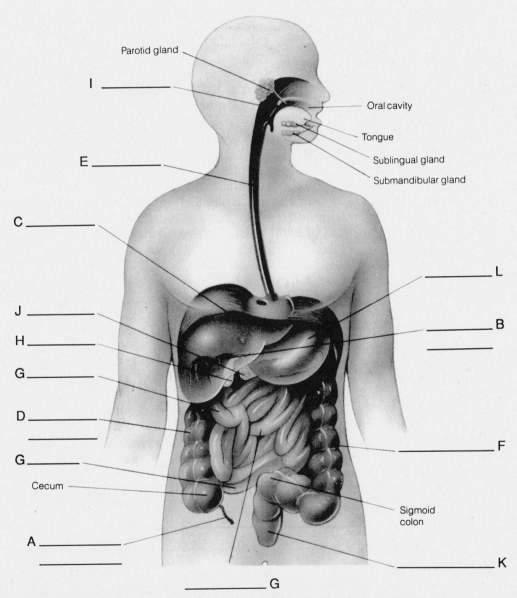

Parotid gland

I _____

Oral cavity

Tongue

Sublingual gland

Submandibular gland

E _____

C _____

L _____

J _____

B _____

H _____

G _____

D _____

F _____

G _____

Cecum

Sigmoid colon

A _____

K _____

_____ G

(Gaudin A.J., Jones K.C.: Human Anatomy and Physiology. Orlando, Harcourt Brace Jovanovich, 1989, p441)

Match the structures on the drawing above to the terms below:

| | | | | | | |
|---|---|---|---|---|---|---|
| G 1. | small intestine | I 5. | pharynx | C 9. | liver |
| G 2. | pancreas | D 6. | ascending colon | B 10. | transverse colon |
| H 3. | esophagus | 7 7. | appendix | H 11. | gallbladder |
| F 4. | descending colon | K 8. | rectum | L 12. | stomach |

141

13. The most common cause of hemorrhage in the abdomen is bleeding from the:

    a. spleen
    b. peritoneum
    c. digestive tract
    d. urinary tract

14. Infections of the abdomen can ultimately spread to the lining of the abdominal cavity. This condition is called:

    a. pleuritis
    b. mesentitis
    c. peritonitis
    d. colitis

15. The superior border of the abdominal cavity is defined by the:

    a. large intestines
    b. liver
    c. diaphragm
    d. peritoneum

16. The pelvic cavity is formed by the pelvic bones and separated from the abdominal cavity by an imaginary plane from the sacrum to the:

    a. umbilicus
    b. diaphragm
    c. pubic symphysis
    d. top of the bladder

17. The lining of the inner abdominal cavity is called the:

    a. pleura
    b. lining abdominis
    c. intima
    d. peritoneum

18. With forced expiration, the upper portion the diaphragm can extend as high as the ___ intercostal space.

    a. 2nd
    b. 4th
    c. 8th
    d. 10th

19. Anteriorly, we can divide the abdomen by two imaginary lines through the _____ into four quadrants.

    a. pelvic bone
    b. umbilicus
    c. xiphoid process
    d. stomach region

20.     The femoral pulse can be palpated halfway between the anterior superior iliac spine of the pelvis and the:

   a.     femur bone
   b.     pubic symphysis
   c.     umbilicus
   d.     top of the pubic hairline

21.     The area just below the xiphoid process is commonly called the:

   a.     epigastrium
   b.     suprapubic area
   c.     periumbilical area
   d.     hypogastric region

22.     The <u>primary</u> and largest artery within the abdomen is the abdominal:

   a.     lilac artery
   b.     mesenteric artery
   c.     aorta
   d.     hepatic artery

23.     There are two distinct pain pathways in the abdomen.   The <u>visceral pathway</u> gives perceptions that are imprecise, while the _____ pathway is perceived more clearly.

   a.     somatic
   b.     peritoneal
   c.     neurogenic
   d.     motor

24.     Food is broken down in the digestive system both mechanically and:

   a.     gaseously
   b.     chemically
   c.     abrasively
   d.     thermally

25.     Aspiration of food is prevented during swallowing by closure of the _____ over the airway.

   a.     cricoid
   b.     vallecula
   c.     epiglottis
   d.     base of the tongue

26. The muscular action that moves food in a coordinated manner through the entire digestive system is called:

    a.  clonic action
    b.  digestive spasm
    c.  bowel constriction
    d.  peristalsis

27. Balloon like blood vessels that can protrude through the lower esophageal wall where they can be subject to erosion from gastric acids and cause bleeding are called esophageal:

    a.  reflux
    b.  diverticuli
    c.  hernia
    d.  varices

28. The stomach contents are normally:

    a.  neutral
    b.  acidic
    c.  alkalotic
    d.  very alkalotic

29. The pain of peptic ulcers is often relieved by the administration of:

    a.  aspirin
    b.  antacids
    c.  acetaminophen
    d.  ibuprofen

30. Which of the following is most likely to aggravate the pain of peptic ulcers?

    a.  milk
    b.  coffee
    c.  meat
    d.  fatty foods

31. Bleeding from the stomach may cause "tarry" stools known as:

    a.  hematemesis
    b.  melana
    c.  diarrhea
    d.  hemafeces

32. Food travels from the stomach directly into the:

    a.  small intestine
    b.  transverse colon
    c.  cecum
    d.  descending colon

33.    The first phase of the small intestine is called the:

    a.    jejunum
    b.    ilium
    c.    duodenum
    d.    cecum

34.    The most common emergency arising from the small intestine is:

    a.    duodenal ulcers
    b.    diverticulitis
    c.    colitis
    d.    appendicitis

35.    The abdominal organ that secretes both digestive enzymes and the hormone insulin to regulate the use of glucose by the body's cells is called the:

    a.    liver
    b.    spleen
    c.    gallbladder
    d.    pancreas

36.    The disease that results from failure of the body to produce a sufficient amount of insulin is called:

    a.    glucosis
    b.    Paget's disease
    c.    hypoglycemia
    d.    diabetes

37.    The most common causes of pancreatitis is excessive _____ consumption and gallstones that block pancreatic block outflow.

    a.    alcohol
    b.    fatty food
    c.    drug
    d.    red meat

38.    The large, solid and soft organ located in the right upper quadrant of the abdomen is the:

    a.    pancreas
    b.    spleen
    c.    kidney
    d.    liver

39.    Filtering out toxins from blood is a major function of the:

    a.    colon
    b.    small intestine
    c.    spleen
    d.    liver

40. Liver disease is often accompanied by _____ skin or mucous membranes.

    a. pale
    b. flushed
    c. jaundiced
    d. cyanotic

41. The organ that stores and concentrates bile produced by the liver is called the:

    a. gallbladder
    b. duodenum
    c. urinary bladder
    d. jejunum

42. Cholecystitis is the major medical emergency related to the:

    a. gallbladder
    b. duodenum
    c. urinary bladder
    d. jejunum

43. Cholecystitis usually occurs when _____, or rocklike concretions, block the exit of bile through the ducts leading to the small intestines.

    a. kidney stones
    b. gallstones
    c. pancreatic stones
    d. liver stones

44. Outpouchings of the inner wall of bowel tissue through the muscle layer of the bowel that may result in painless lower GI bleeding are called:

    a. aneurysms
    b. hernias
    c. diverticuli
    d. ulcers

45. Patients with severe diarrhea will develop:

    a. bowel obstruction
    b. necrosis of the colon
    c. ischemia of the bowel
    d. dehydration and hypovolemia

46. A childhood condition occurring when the peristaltic action of the bowel <u>telescopes</u> one portion of the intestine into another resulting in obstruction of the bowel is called:

    a. intussusception
    b. peristaltic obstruction
    c. diverticulosis
    d. incarcerated hernia

47. A condition that starts with umbilical pain that then localizes in the right lower quadrant of the abdomen and is associated with fever, nausea and vomiting is highly suggestive of:

    a. appendicitis
    b. ectopic pregnancy
    c. colitis
    d. cholecystitis

48. The condition caused by ballooning of the veins in the rectal area that can burst and result in rectal bleeding is called:

    a. varices
    b. rectal aneurysms
    c. hemorrhoids
    d. venous hernias

49. The primary organ of the urinary system that is responsible for fluid and electrolyte regulation and filtering toxins from the blood is called the:

    a. bladder
    b. urethra
    c. kidney
    d. ureter

50. The organ of the urinary system that is responsible for storing urine prior to excretion is called the:

    a. bladder
    b. urethra
    c. kidney
    d. ureter

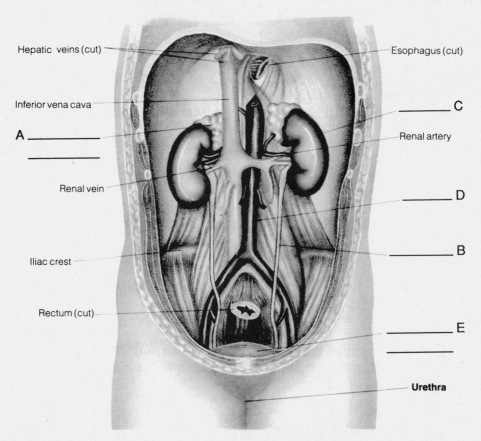

Hepatic veins (cut)

Esophagus (cut)

Inferior vena cava

C

A

Renal artery

Renal vein

D

B

Iliac crest

Rectum (cut)

E

**Urethra**

(Gaudin A.J., Jones K.C.: Human Anatomy and Physiology. Orlando, Harcourt, Brace, Jovanovich, 1989, p647)

Match the structures on the drawing above to the terms below:

B  51. ureters

D  54. aorta

C  52. kidneys

A  55. adrenal gland

E  53. urinary bladder

56.     Absence of urine output, altered mental state, seizures, tachycardia, deep and rapid respirations, pallor, congestive heart failure and pulmonary edema best describe:

    a.      acute urinary retention
    b.      renal failure
    c.      pylonephritis
    d.      cystitis

57.    Infections of the urinary bladder occur more often in:

    a.    children
    b.    men
    c.    women
    d.    newborns

58.    A condition usually caused by obstruction of the urethra characterized by suprapubic pain and a feeling of distress, common in elderly men, is called:

    a.    cystitis
    b.    pyelonephritis
    c.    acute urinary retention
    d.    nephritis

59.    Tearing abdominal pain and/or back pain associated with a wide palpable pulsating mass in the midline in the upper abdomen best describes:

    a.    abdominal aortic aneurysm
    b.    dissecting aneurysm
    c.    berry aneurysm
    d.    peptic ulcer

60.    A patient who is lying with his knees drawn up and who has shallow breaths, local or diffuse abdominal tenderness or guarding, hypovolemia, rapid pulse and perhaps lowered blood pressure best describes someone with:

    a.    acute urinary retention
    b.    an acute abdomen
    c.    acute pylonephritis
    d.    acute cystitis

61.    When palpating the abdomen of a patient with abdominal pain, you should begin:

    a.    at the location of pain
    b.    away from the area of pain
    c.    at the lower margin of the abdomen
    d.    at the upper margin of the abdomen

62.    The two organs most commonly injured as a result of blunt abdominal trauma are the:

    a.    stomach and pancreas
    b.    small and large intestines
    c.    spleen and liver
    d.    kidneys and bladder

63.     The process in which organs or vessels continue to move forward and tear at a point of attachment during a sudden cessation of motion in a fall or auto collision best describes what mechanism of injury?

    a.    contrecoup
    b.    deceleration
    c.    penetrating
    d.    velocity tears

64.     What two organs in the abdomen are most likely to be injured because of the mechanism of injury described in the previous question?

    a.    liver and kidneys
    b.    bladder and stomach
    c.    ureters and urethra
    d.    esophagus and pancreas

65.     The factor that most affects the extent of injury due to gunshot wounds is the:

    a.    mass of the bullet
    b.    velocity of the bullet
    c.    shape of the bullet
    d.    none of the above

66.     Which of the following is a late sign of hypovolemic shock that may be noted with intraabdominal hemorrhage?

    a.    delayed capillary refill
    b.    tachycardia
    c.    pale skin
    d.    hypotension

67.     The primary wound care for an evisceration should include a:

    a.    dry sterile dressing
    b.    moistened or airtight dressing
    c.    petroleum jelly dressing
    d.    Teflon gauze dressing

68.     Penetrating objects impaled in the abdomen should be:

    a.    left alone
    b.    carefully removed
    c.    stabilized in place
    d.    cut off a skin level

69.    Generally speaking, patients with abdominal trauma should be placed in the position of comfort:

    a.    sitting upright
    b.    lying on their side
    c.    supine with hips and knees flexed
    d.    prone with knees flexed

70.    If a rape patient recounts the details of the assault, you should:

    a.    paraphrase the statement on your record
    b.    ignore it since it is police business
    c.    record the exact statement
    d.    record it on a separate document

71.    If a rape patient should desire to take a shower prior to coming to the hospital, you should:

    a.    advise against it to preserve evidence
    b.    respect their wishes and wait for the patient
    c.    advise them to shower but not to douche
    d.    forcibly restrain them to preserve evidence

72.    If parts of the male and female genitalia are completely avulsed or amputated in an assault you should:

    a.    leave them on the scene for evidence
    b.    wrap in gauze and plastic bag and place on ice
    c.    place in saline solution
    d.    reattach them in their normal position

## Case Histories

### Case History #1

You find a 48 year old male responsive to verbal stimuli. He appears pale, sweaty and cool to the touch. His wife advises you that he fainted on the bathroom floor of his apartment 20 minutes ago and regained consciousness about 5 minutes later. He becomes extremely dizzy when placed in the sitting position. His vital signs are blood pressure 78/60, pulse 140 and thready, and respirations 24 and shallow. He has a history of a heart attack and high blood pressure. He complains of tenderness in the epigastric region of his abdomen, and his abdomen is rigid.

73.    He advises you that his last bowel movement had a black and tarry consistency. What do you suspect is the primary problem?

    a.    upper gastrointestinal bleeding
    b.    abdominal aortic aneurysm
    c.    lower gastrointestinal bleeding
    d.    hepatitis

74. Based on his vital signs you suspect _____ hypovolemic shock.

    a. early
    b. compensated
    c. late
    d. moderate

75. His dizziness when sitting up is probably caused by:

    a. vasodilation
    b. orthostatic hypotension
    c. tachycardia
    d. ischemia to the heart

76. The management of this patient would include:

    a. nonrebreather mask and PASG
    b. nonrebreather mask and no PASG
    c. nasal cannula and PASG
    d. nasal cannula and no PASG

---

### Case History #2

You find a 63 year old woman in her bed at home. She is responsive to painful but not verbal stimuli and is confused and disoriented. She is extremely jaundiced and has a distended abdomen that is tender in the upper right quadrant. Her daughter states that she has had loss of appetite, nausea and vomiting over the last two days. Her vital signs are blood pressure 190/110, pulse 100 and regular, and respirations 24 and deep.

---

77. Based on the history and physical findings, which two problems are the most likely causes of her condition?

    a. hepatitis and cirrhosis
    b. pancreatitis and colitis
    c. appendicitis and diverticulitis
    d. gastritis and esophagitis

78. Which of the following is a common cause of these conditions?

    a. smoking
    b. alcoholism
    c. hypertension
    d. dehydration

79. Based on the level of consciousness and the other signs, what complication of this condition might the patient be experiencing?

    a. pancreatic failure
    b. ruptured appendix
    c. esophageal bleeding
    d. liver failure

---

### Case History #3

You find a 17 year old boy lying in bed with his knees drawn up and immobile and in extreme distress. He states that he has severe abdominal pain that began 24 hours ago in his umbilical region and is now localized in his right lower quadrant. His has tenderness in his right lower quadrant and his abdomen is very rigid. When you remove your fingertips during palpation, he experiences diffuse pain throughout his abdomen. He has fever, nausea, and vomiting. His vital signs are blood pressure 110/70, pulse 110 and regular, and respirations 24 and shallow.

---

80. Based on the signs and symptoms, what do you suspect is the underlying condition?

    a. colitis
    b. appendicitis
    c. gastritis
    d. intussuception

81. Based on the rigid abdomen and response to palpation, what complication do you suspect?

    a. severe hemorrhage
    b. ischemic bowel
    c. peritonitis
    d. obstruction of the bowel

82. His initial umbilical pain was most likely _____ pain.

    a. visceral
    b. ischemic
    c. somatic
    d. colic

---

### Case History #4

You find a 70 year old male who is responsive to verbal stimuli on the floor of his living room. His wife states that he woke up with severe "tearing" abdominal pain radiating to his back and collapsed on the floor on the way to the bathroom. He skin is pale, sweaty and cool, and he has a pulsatile abdominal mass on the midline of his abdomen. His vital signs are blood pressure 120/100, pulse 110 and thready, and respirations 26 and shallow.

---

83.    Based on the presenting signs and symptoms, you suspect:

     a.    gastrointestinal bleeding
     b.    diverticulitis
     c.    appendicitis
     d.    abdominal aortic aneurysm

84.    His physical findings and vital signs would suggest that he is in a
                   _____ stage of hypovolemic shock.

     a.    decompensated
     b.    compensated
     c.    late
     d.    final

---

### Case History #5

At the scene of a frontend collision you find an 18 year old female who was the driver of a car. She is complaining of severe left upper quadrant abdominal pain, with pain in the left shoulder. She is alert and oriented and has delayed capillary refill and pale and sweaty skin. Her vital signs are blood pressure 80/64, pulse 132 and regular, and respirations 28 and shallow.

---

85.    Based on the presenting signs and symptoms, you suspect a ruptured:

     a.    liver
     b.    spleen
     c.    stomach
     d.    bowel

86.    The term used to describe the pain in her left shoulder is:

     a.    rebound
     b.    referred
     c.    relocated
     d.    radiating

87.    Based on the presenting signs and symptoms, the management of this patient should include:

     a.    PASG
     b.    oxygen via Venturi mask
     c.    sitting position
     d.    oropharyngeal airway

---

### Case History #6

You respond to a shooting at a bar and find a 48 year old male with a small round wound in the center of his abdomen. A bystander states that he was shot 5 minutes ago with a hunting rifle from a distance of 10 feet. He is alert and experiencing severe abdominal pain. His vital signs are blood pressure 170/100, pulse 90 and regular, and respirations 20 and deep.

---

88. Based on the information about the shooting, you would suspect the zone of injury within the abdominal cavity to be:

    a. about the diameter of the bullet
    b. smaller that the diameter of the bullet
    c. slightly larger than the diameter of the bullet
    d. much larger than the diameter of the bullet

89. You would expect the exit wound to be _____ in relation to the entrance wound.

    a. smaller
    b. larger
    c. the same size
    d. pinpoint

---

### Case History #7

You respond to an assault and find a 19 year old female who states that she was raped and sodomized. Her clothing is torn and strewn throughout the room, and there is blood and secretions on her face, abdomen and perineum.

---

90. The management of this patient should include:

    a. collecting specific facts about the rape
    b. washing the body fluids away to prevent infection
    c. focusing on injuries and psychological care
    d. examine all of the orifices with a gloved hand

91. The preservation of evidence is the responsibility of:

    a. everyone coming into contact with the patient
    b. the police
    c. the physician and nurses
    d. the district attorney

155

Skill Performance Sheet

**Applying an Evisceration Dressing and Bandage**

Student Name_____          Date_____

| Performance Standard | Performed | Failed |
|---|---|---|
| MOISTENED DRESSING TYPE | | |
| Moisten multitrauma dressing | \| | \| |
| Apply to exposed bowel | \| | \| |
| Cover with dry dressing | \| | \| |
| Tape in place | \| | \| |
| PLASTIC WRAP OR ALUMINUM FOIL TYPE | | |
| Apply wrap to bowel | \| | \| |
| Tape border completely to create airtight seal | \| | \| |

Comments_____

_____

_____

_____

Instructor _____          Circle One:   Pass   Fail

## Chapter 9

## SOFT TISSUE INJURIES

1. The surface or outermost layer of the skin is called the:

   a. subcutaneous layer
   b. fascia
   c. epidermis
   d. dermis

2. The epidermis contains a special pigment that helps protect us from the sun's radiation and contributes to the color of the skin called:

   a. melanin
   b. keratan
   c. surfactant
   d. sebum

3. When blood flow to the skin is reduced (as a result of vasoconstriction in hypovolemic shock or in cold temperatures) the skin may appear:

   a. red
   b. cyanotic
   c. pale
   d. mottled

4. The layer of the skin that is composed of dense connective tissue that contains the nerves, blood vessels, sweat and sebaceous glands, and hair follicles is called:

   a. subcutaneous layer
   b. fascia
   c. epidermis
   d. dermis

5. If the dermis is completely damaged, as in third degree burns, there will be _____ sensory perception.

   a. increased
   b. extremely painful
   c. no
   d. tingling

6. As skin continues into a body orifice, it changes its character. The keratinized layer of the epidermis is absent and is replaced by:

   a. mucous membranes
   b. connective tissue
   c. muscle tissue
   d. fatty tissue

7.   Beneath the skin is a layer of fat and connective tissue called the:

    a.   mucosa
    b.   subcutaneous layer
    c.   subdermal layer
    d.   peritoneum

Match the description in column B with the type of wound in column A.

| Column A | | Column B | |
|---|---|---|---|
| 8. | E contusion | a. | tearing away of the skin's surface |
| 9. | C abrasion | b. | wound caused by a sharp instrument being driven through the skin |
| 10. | D laceration | | |
| 11. | A avulsion | c. | scraping of the surface of the skin or mucous membrane |
| 12. | B puncture | d. | a tearing of the skin or other soft tissues |
| | | e. | bruising of the skin |

13.   In general, impaled objects should be:

    a.   stabilized in place
    b.   carefully removed
    c.   repositioned to facilitate bandaging
    d.   left alone

14.   Objects impaled in the cheek should be:

    a.   stabilized in place
    b.   carefully removed
    c.   repositioned to facilitate bandaging
    d.   left alone

15.   What vessels are likely to promote air embolism when severed?

    a.   arteries in the head
    b.   veins in the neck and upper chest
    c.   capillaries in the chest
    d.   arteries in the chest

16. When a neck vein is severed, you should:

    a. apply a Teflon dressing and sit the patient upright
    b. apply an airtight dressing and place the patient supine
    c. apply a saline dressing and place the patient on his or her side
    d. apply a multitrauma dressing and place the patient prone

Match the description in column B with the type of bandage or dressing in column A.

| Column A | | Column B |
|---|---|---|
| C 17. | multitrauma | a. used as a sling or cravat bandage |
| A 18. | triangular | b. aluminum foil, plastic wrap or petroleum gauze |
| D 19. | self-adherent | c. large dressing used for massive abrasions or burns |
| B 20. | occlusive | d. allows elastic pressure for arterial bleeding |

21. The first concern for a patient with injuries to the face and neck is the:

    a. cervical spine
    b. airway
    c. eye
    d. brain

Match the description in column B with the appropriate facial bone in column A.

| Column A | | Column B |
|---|---|---|
| B 22. | mandible | a. connects maxilla, frontal and temporal bones |
| A 23. | zygoma | b. bone of the lower jaw |
| D 24. | frontal | c. bone of the upper jaw |
| C 25. | maxilla | d. bone of the forehead |

26.    The categorization of midface facial fractures into three groups in relation to the level and instability of the facial bones is called:

    a.    Le Fort fractures
    b.    Cushing's fractures
    c.    Colles' fractures
    d.    Homan's fractures

27.    When the teeth are not aligned properly or the patient is unable to close his mouth, it may suggest a fracture of the:

    a.    zygoma
    b.    frontal bone
    c.    orbit
    d.    mandible

28.    Fractures of the jaw may cause collapse and obstruction of the airway. If this is encountered, you should:

    a.    perform a head tilt-neck lift
    b.    pull the tongue and lower jaw forward
    c.    perform a tracheostomy
    d.    transport and do nothing

29.    Patients with facial injuries (where cervical spine injuries are not suspected) and associated bleeding in the airway should be placed in the _____ position.

    a.    supine
    b.    prone
    c.    lateral recumbent
    d.    Trendelenberg

30.    Complete and deep avulsions of the facial skin should be treated by placing a _____ dressing directly over the wound.

    a.    petroleum jelly
    b.    aluminum foil
    c.    moistened
    d.    Surgipad

31.    The nose is divided in halves by the cartilagenous structure called the:

    a.    nares
    b.    palate
    c.    septum
    d.    pharynx

32. Ninety percent of all nosebleeds occur in the _____ portion of the nose.

    a. anterior
    b. middle
    c. posterior
    d. external

33. Control of bleeding in the nose is initially attempted by direct pressure:

    a. with two fingers on the upper nose
    b. with two fingers over the nostrils
    c. on the internal surface of the nose
    d. over the cheek area

34. If nosebleeding is not controlled by direct pressure, a pressure point can be used:

    a. under the upper lip
    b. on the forehead
    c. on the cheek
    d. on the lower rim of the orbit

35. The most common cause of nosebleeds is:

    a. fractures of the face
    b. self-induced exploration of the nostrils
    c. high blood pressure
    d. inflammation of the nasal mucosa

36. Serious uncontrolled nosebleeds usually originate from the _____ portion of the nose.

    a. anterior
    b. middle
    c. posterior
    d. external

37. The eye is a globular structure filled with a gel-like fluid called the:

    a. vitreous humor
    b. mucus
    c. peritoneal fluid
    d. plasma

38. The collection of bones that surround the eye is commonly called the:

    a. occular bones
    b. orbit
    c. perioccular bones
    d. acetabular

# Chapter 9

39. The white outer layer of the eye, which is composed of a tough, fibrous, and opaque (not transparent to light) protective membrane is called the:

    a. cornea
    b. retina
    c. lens
    d. sclera

40. The pigmented or colored portion of the eye that regulates the diameter of the pupil is called the:

    a. retina
    b. iris
    c. cornea
    d. macula

41. Anatomically the eye can be divided into an anterior and posterior chamber by the:

    a. lens
    b. conjuctiva
    c. retina
    d. macula

42. When drainage of the aqueous humor is obstructed, pressure builds up and causes a condition known as:

    a. retinitis
    b. glaucoma
    c. cataracts
    d. aqueous tension

43. Tears are secreted by the _____ located at the superolateral surface of each eyeball.

    a. mucous cells
    b. ocular duct
    c. lacrimal glands
    d. cornea

44. General principles for treating eye injuries include:

    a. always irrigate and apply firm pressure
    b. avoid pressure and cover both eyes
    c. never treat in the field
    d. use petroleum gauze and never cover both eyes

45.    The best method for removing foreign bodies of the eye in the field is:

    a.     with the use of suction cups
    b.     irrigation
    c.     with the use of a cotton tip applicator
    d.     by rapid eyelid movement

46.    A cotton tip applicator should never be used to remove foreign bodies of the:

    a.     cornea
    b.     eyelid
    c.     sclera
    d.     lacrimal gland

47.    Impaled objects in the eyeball should be treated by:

    a.     pulling them out with a gloved hand
    b.     repositioning them to facilitate bandaging
    c.     stabilizing them in place
    d.     leaving them alone

48.    Chemical burns to the eye are treated by:

    a.     bandaging the affected eye
    b.     irrigating with water or sterile saline
    c.     irrigating with an alkaline solution
    d.     rapid transport without field treatment

49.    Light injuries caused by overexposure to too much infrared light from the sun or to ultraviolet light from arc welding is treated by:

    a.     placing moist patches over the eyes
    b.     taping the eyes closed
    c.     placing a cup over the eyes
    d.     irrigating the eyes

50.    The term given to this traumatically induced spasm of the iris muscle is:

    a.     traumatic iritis
    b.     cataracts
    c.     glaucoma
    d.     spasmotic iritis

51.    An extruded eyeball should be managed by:

    a.     replacing it in the eye socket
    b.     covering it with a dry 4x4 bandage and a patch
    c.     covering it with a moist dressing and a cup
    d.     irrigation during transport

52.    A highly infectious condition characterized by an itching and a pink or red appearance to the white portion of the eye is called:

      a.     conjuctivitis
      b.     retinitis
      c.     scleritis
      d.     glauoma

53.    The outer visible flap of the ear is called the:

      a.     pinna
      b.     malleus
      c.     nares
      d.     vestibule

54.    The middle ear communicates with the nasopharynx via the:

      a.     semicircular canal
      b.     cochlea
      c.     eustachian tube
      d.     vestibule

55.    Other than hearing, the middle ear also contributes to control of:

      a.     voice transmission
      b.     heat exchange
      c.     balance and position
      d.     fluid excretion

56.    Blood or clear fluid flowing from the ear should always be considered as a possible sign of:

      a.     skull fracture
      b.     eardrum rupture
      c.     cochlea injury
      d.     overhydration

57.    <u>Incomplete</u> avulsed parts of the auricle are treated by:

      a.     replacing them in anatomical position and bandaging
      b.     removing them and storing them in saline solution
      c.     placing an ice pack over the site and transporting
      d.     irrigating with Betadine and alcohol solution

58.    The rupture of the eardrum due to changes in altitude and pressure is a type of:

      a.     tympanic syndrome
      b.     barotrauma
      c.     the bends
      d.     pneumotympanic rupture

59.  The presence of subcutaneous emphysema in the neck region is highly suggestive of:

a.  air embolism
b.  chronic lung disease
c.  tearing or fractures of the airway
d.  barotrauma

60.  Dyspnea, cyanosis, stridor and difficulty in talking associated with trauma to the neck is highly suggestive of trauma to the:

a.  pharynx
b.  larynx
c.  bronchi
d.  respiratory muscles

## Case Histories

| Case History #1 |
| --- |
| You find a 28 year old male lying on the livingroom floor of his apartment and bleeding profusely from the face.  His wife states that he tripped and fell on a glass coffee table.  You note upon examination that he is in severe respiratory distress and has a large fragment of glass impaled in his left cheek that projects into his oral cavity. |

61.  The greatest <u>immediate</u> risk with this patient is:

a.  aspiration and airway obstruction
b.  bleeding to death
c.  neurogenic shock due to panic
d.  severe infection

62.  Your first action should be to:

a.  stabilize the glass with a stacked dressing and transport immediately
b.  turn the patient into the prone position and transport immediately
c.  remove the glass and hold direct pressure on the inside and outside of the wound
d.  place a suction catheter in the mouth and continuously suction during transport

---

### Case History #2

You respond to a construction site and find a 40 year old male in severe pain and holding his hand over his eye. Bystanders state that he was accidently stabbed in the eye socket with a sharp pipe. Upon close examination, you note that his left eye is completely avulsed and hanging approximately 3 inches out of the socket.

---

63.     The immediate care of the eye should consist of applying a:

      a.     dry 4x4 dressing
      b.     moist dressing
      c.     petroleum dressing
      d.     Betadine-soaked dressing

64.     After applying the dressing, the eyeball can be stabilized with:

      a.     adhesive tape
      b.     a cup and bandage
      c.     a Kling bandage
      d.     a stacked dressing

---

### Case History #3

You arrive at the site of a train and car collision and find a 19 year old male who is responsive to verbal stimuli. You observe that he has suffered bilateral amputations of the lower thigh, just above the knee, which are bleeding profusely. (These questions include a partial review of Chapter 5.)

---

65.     After failed attempts to control bleeding with direct pressure, you apply bilateral pressure point at which of the following locations?

      a.     lateral aspect of the thigh between the hip bone and the iliac crest
      b.     midline over the pubic symphysis, just below the umbilicus
      c.     midway between the pubic symphysis and the iliac crest
      d.     midline on the posterior thigh between the hip and the knee

66.     The pressure point fails to control the bleeding, and you decide to apply a tourniquet at the:

      a.     groin region at the site of the femoral pulse
      b.     upper thigh region, 2 inches below the groin
      c.     mid-thigh region
      d.     a few inches above the wound

67.     The amputated parts should be managed by:

    a.    placing them in a plastic bag and then placing the plastic bag on ice
    b.    soaking them in saline solution and placing the legs directly on ice
    c.    wrapping them in an occlusive dressing to maintain the moisture
    d.    wrapping them in a multitrauma dressing to maintain sterility

---

### Case History #4

You respond to an automobile collision and find a 38 year woman who has been thrown through the windshield.  You note a deep laceration in the left lower neck region just above the clavicle with venous bleeding.

---

68.     A major potential complication specific to this type of neck wound is:

    a.    brain infection
    b.    air embolism
    c.    tendon laceration
    d.    carotid thrombus

69.     The neck wound should be managed with a(n):

    a.    sterile 4x4 dressing
    b.    Kling wrap around the neck
    c.    multitrauma dressing
    d.    airtight dressing

70.     The best position of transport for this patient is:

    a.    sitting upright (90 degree angle)
    b.    the semireclining position (45 degree angle)
    c.    the Trendelenberg position (hips and legs elevated)
    d.    the supine position

---

### Case History #5

A 14 year old is found at the bottom of a stairwell with a large avulsion of the scalp.  The 6 inch flap of scalp is folded posterior, exposing a large area of subcutaneous tissue.  It is attached to the remaining skin with a 1 inch segment of tissue.  The patient is alert and oriented and has no disability findings, but you note clear liquid escaping from the ear.

---

71.    The management of the avulsed part should include:

      a.     disconnecting the flap from skin and storing it in a bag of ice
      b.     rinsing the tissue and placing it in the normal anatomical position
      c.     bandaging it as it is found with a Kling bandage
      d.     placing an ice pack on the scalp and bandaging it in place

72.    The clear liquid escaping from the ear suggests the possibility of a:

      a.     basilar skull fracture
      b.     eardrum rupture
      c.     wound infection
      d.     brainstem laceration

73.    The leaking fluid should be managed by:

      a.     the application of ice over the ear
      b.     packing the ear with gauze
      c.     applying a loose dressing
      d.     applying a cup over the ear

---

### Case History #6

A scuba diver complains of a severe earache after decending 50 feet below the surface. He states that he had a slight cold and congestion for 3 days prior to the dive.

---

74.    Based on the history, what injury do you suspect?

      a.     the bends
      b.     barotrauma to the eardrum
      c.     ruptured cochlea
      d.     severe middle ear infection

75.    This problem is due to a clogged:

      a.     external ear
      b.     middle ear
      c.     eustachian tube
      d.     cochlea

---

### Case History #7

You find the driver of a frontend automobile collision in severe respiratory distress. Upon physical exam, you note stridor, accessory muscle use and subcutaneous emphysema on the neck and upper chest.

---

76.  The most likely diagnosis based on the above findings is:

     a.  tension pneumothorax
     b.  ruptured trachea or larynx
     c.  traumatic asphyxia
     d.  flail chest

77.  If this patient were to show signs of complete obstruction of the airway, what would your actions be?

     a.  positive pressure and rapid transport
     b.  abdominal or chest thrusts
     c.  immediate back blows between the scapula
     d.  finger sweeps followed by positive pressure ventilation

Skill Performance Sheet

**Basic Bandage Application**

Student Name_____          Date_____

| Performance Standard | Performed | Failed |
| --- | --- | --- |
| Take universal precautions (gloves, goggles) | | |
| Apply dressing over wound | | |
| Circle area and anchor bandage | | |
| Begin circular attachment of bandage covering the previous layer by 50% each time | | |
| Continue past the dressing and secure bandage in place | | |
| Elevate the affected part | | |
| Check distal pulse | | |

Comments_____

_____

_____

_____

Instructor _____          Circle One:  Pass  Fail

Skill Performance Sheet

**Stabilizing an Impaled Object**

Student Name_____     Date_____

| Performance Standard | Performed | Failed |
|---|---|---|
| Take universal precautions (gloves, goggles) | | |
| EMT #1 stabilizes object with hand | | |
| Place stacked multitrauma dressing on both sides of the object approximately half up | | |
| Tape across the dressings in both directions to provide support | | |
| Check to establish stability | | |
| Reinforce as needed | | |

Comments_____

_____

_____

_____

Instructor _____     Circle One:   Pass   Fail

## Chapter 10

## MUSCULOSKELETAL SYSTEM

1.    The axial skeleton consists of the:

  a. skull, spine, ribs and sternum
  b. pelvis and lower extremities
  c. upper extremities and clavicles
  d. the joints of the body

2.    A softer precursor of bone that is present throughout the body and persists at sites of bone growth and at joints to provide a smooth, friction-free surface is called:

  a. ligaments
  b. tendons
  c. cartilage
  d. fascia

3.    Connective bands of tissue that attach bone to bone and maintain the stability of joints are called:

  a. ligaments
  b. tendons
  c. cartilage
  d. fascia

4.    Thin bands of tissue that attach muscle to bone and initiate movement of joints are called:

  a. ligaments
  b. tendons
  c. cartilage
  d. fascia

Match the bones in column B to the appropriate type of bone in column A.

| Column A | | Column B | |
|---|---|---|---|
| C 5. | short bone | a. | femur |
| D 6. | irregular bone | b. | sternum |
| A 7. | long bone | c. | metatarsal bone |
| B 8. | flat bone | d. | vertebra |

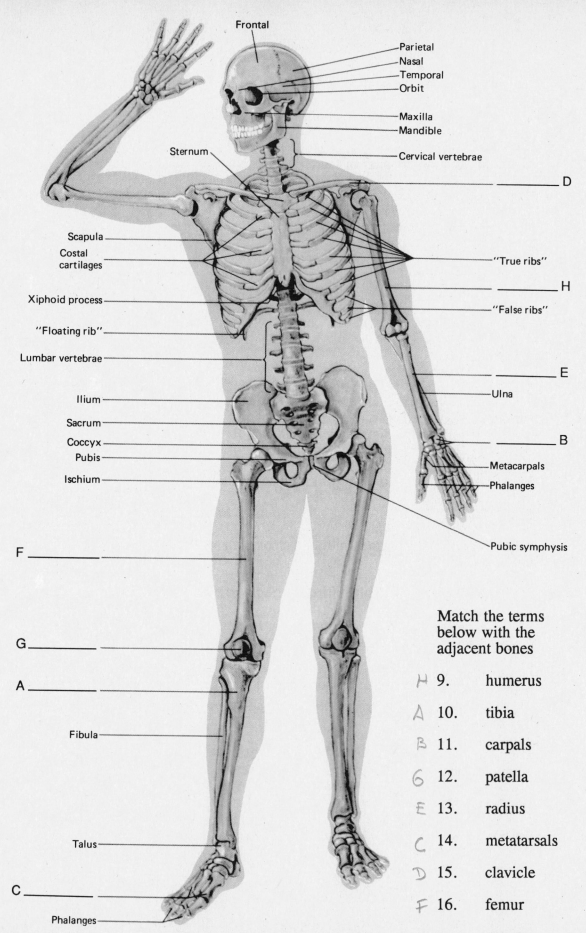

Frontal
Parietal
Nasal
Temporal
Orbit
Maxilla
Mandible
Cervical vertebrae
D
Sternum
Scapula
Costal cartilages
"True ribs"
H
Xiphoid process
"False ribs"
"Floating rib"
Lumbar vertebrae
E
Ulna
Ilium
Sacrum
Coccyx
B
Pubis
Ischium
Metacarpals
Phalanges
Pubic symphysis
F
G
A
Fibula
Talus
C
Phalanges

Match the terms below with the adjacent bones

H  9.   humerus
A  10.  tibia
B  11.  carpals
G  12.  patella
E  13.  radius
C  14.  metatarsals
D  15.  clavicle
F  16.  femur

(Solomon EP, Phillips GA:  Understanding Human Anatomy and Physiology.  Philadelphia, WB Saunders, 1987, p75)

17.  The portion of bone responsible for the production of red blood cells is:

   a.  spongy bone
   b.  periosteum
   c.  red marrow
   d.  epiphysis

18.  The fibrous membrane that covers bone except at the articular surfaces (joints) is:

   a.  marrow
   b.  cartilage
   c.  periosteum
   d.  epiphyseal plate

Match the structures in column B to the appropriate type of muscle in column A.

| Column A | | Column B | |
|---|---|---|---|
| A 19. | smooth | a. | blood vessel |
| C 20. | cardiac | b. | biceps |
| B 21. | skeletal | c. | heart |

22.  The elbow is an example of a _____ joint.

   a.  hinged
   b.  ball and socket
   c.  fused
   d.  gliding

23.  Displacement of bones in a joint from their normal anatomical position is called a:

   a.  compression injury
   b.  dislocation
   c.  sprain
   d.  strain

24.  The stretching or tearing of a ligament is called a:

   a.  compression injury
   b.  dislocation
   c.  sprain
   d.  strain

25. When a bone is diseased as the result of cancer or osteoporosis, fractures may result from relatively minor mechanisms of injury. These are called _____ fractures.

    a. stress
    b. compression
    c. simple
    d. pathological

26. Fractures that result from continued pounding and overuse that often occur with joggers or runners are called _____ fractures.

    a. stress
    b. compression
    c. simple
    d. pathological

Match the description in column B with the type of fracture in column A.

| Column A | | Column B | |
|---|---|---|---|
| E | 27. closed | a. | caused by a twisting force |
| A | 28. spiral | b. | fracture associated with a break in the skin |
| G | 29. transverse | | |
| | | c. | fragment of bone due to a forceful muscle contraction |
| H | 30. greenstick | | |
| I | 31. impacted | e. | fracture without a break in skin |
| C | 32. avulsion | | |
| | | f. | multiple fragments of bone at the fracture site |
| F | 33. comminuted | | |
| | | g. | fracture perpendicular to bone produced by direct force |
| | | h. | incomplete fracture common in children |
| | | i. | fracture resulting in bone driven into bone |

34. The term used to describe the sensation felt during palpation that is created by the grating of bone ends together is:

    a. friction rub
    b. Homan's sign
    c. rhonchi
    d. crepitus

35. A joint locked in a deformed position following an injury is highly suggestive of a:

   a.   sprain
   b.   dislocation
   c.   strain
   d.   spiral fracture

36. The 5 P's that may indicate vascular or nerve injury in a fractured extremity include pain, pulselessness, pallor, paresthesia (numbness or tingling) and:

   a.   paralysis
   b.   priapism
   c.   purple skin
   d.   palpitations

37. Bladder, rectal and urethral injuries are commonly associated with fracture of the:

   a.   femur
   b.   lumbar spine
   c.   pelvis
   d.   hip

38. Fat can sometimes be released following a fracture and cause:

   a.   a tumor
   b.   hypoglycemia
   c.   an embolism
   d.   inflammation

Match the type of force in column B to the appropriate mechanism of injury in column A.

| Column A | Column B |
| --- | --- |
| C 39.  bumper striking a tibia causing a transverse fracture at the site of impact | a.  twisting force |
| | b.  indirect force along bone's axis |
| A 40.  an ice skater fracturing the tibia while performing a spin due to the blade being trapped in the ice | c.  direct force |
| B 41.  a humerus fracture after a fall on an outstretched hand | |

*Chapter 10*

42.     The most common sign or symptom of a fracture is:

      a.     discoloration
      b.     deformity
      c.     pain
      d.     swelling

43.     Which of the following is a major cause of deformity following a fracture?

      a.     the pulling force of opposing muscles
      b.     ecchymosis at the site of injury
      c.     obstruction of an artery
      d.     nerve paralysis in the extremity

44.     Absence of capillary refill in a single extremity is highly suggestive of:

      a.     hypovolemic shock secondary to severe blood loss and vasoconstriction
      b.     vascular compromise due to a fracture or dislocation
      c.     spinal shock causing vasoconstriction to one side of the body
      d.     cardiac tamponade causing poor cardiac output through the aorta

45.     Which of the following types of fractures are most likely to result in stability and the ability for motion of the affected extremity?

      a.     transverse and spiral
      b.     impacted and greenstick
      c.     compound and oblique
      d.     pathologic and comminuted

46.     A primary rule of fracture management is to splint the fracture site and the:

      a.     surrounding tissues
      b.     distal extremity
      c.     adjacent joints
      d.     proximal extremity

Match the type of splint in column B with the descriptions in column A.

Column A                                                    Column B

*C*   47.   made of padded cardboard,              a.   traction splint
            wood, metal or plastic
                                                   b.   pillow splint
*F*   48.   environmental temperature
            can impair function                    c.   rigid splint

*E*   49.   can be shaped and molded               d.   sling and swathe
            to conform to an extremity
                                                   e.   wire ladder splint
*B*   50.   best ankle splint
                                                   f.   air splint
*D*   51.   can be made from triangular
            bandages

*A*   52.   best splint for femur
            fracture

53.   The bone that can be palpated on the anterior upper chest region that extends
      from the sternum to the shoulder region is called the:

      a.   scapula
      b.   glenoid
      c.   olecranon
      (d.)  clavicle

54.   Injuries to the shoulder, humerus, scapula and clavicle are best treated with
      a(n):

      a.   pillow splint
      (b.)  sling and swathe
      c.   rigid splint
      d.   air splint

55.   Which of the following fractures (in and of itself) is highly suggestive of a
      severe mechanism of injury and a likelihood of underlying chest trauma?

      a.   clavicle
      b.   humerus
      (c.)  scapula
      d.   shoulder

56.   The most common mechanism of injury for the upper extremity is a:

      a.   direct blow
      (b.)  fall on an outstretched hand
      c.   twisting force
      d.   hyperextension injury

57. In shoulder dislocations, the humerus is usually displaced:

    a.  laterally
    b.  medially
    c.  anteriorly
    d.  posteriorly

58. In most shoulder dislocations, the patient will resist movement:

    a.  toward the chest (adduction)
    b.  away from the chest (abduction)
    c.  rotating externally
    d.  both b and c

59. Vascular compromise resulting from shoulder dislocations can be evaluated by palpating the _____ artery.

    a.  popliteal
    b.  dorsalis pedis
    c.  radial
    d.  humeral

60. When treating a fracture of the humerus the sling and swathe can be augmented by a ____ inch rigid splint placed between the medial side of the humerus and the chest wall.

    a.  3
    b.  5
    c.  9
    d   18

61. Children between 1 and 4 years old are susceptible to dislocations of the elbow due to sudden traction on an outstretched arm. This condition is known as:

    a.  elbow hyperextension
    b.  Colles' fracture
    c.  boxer's injury
    d.  nursemaid's elbow

62. A complication of elbow dislocation where the fingers become contracted and dysfunctional is called _____ contracture.

    a.  Volkmann's
    b.  Homan's
    c.  Colles'
    d.  phalange

63.    Angulated elbow fractures or dislocations are best immobilized by a(n):

   a.    pillow splint on the medial side of the arm
   b.    bridge splint from the radius to the humerus
   c.    sling and swathe
   d.    air splint extending from the wrist to the
         axilla

64.    The bones of the forearm include the radius and the:

   a.    humerus
   b.    fibula
   c.    manubrium
   d.    ulna

65.    Fractures of the wrist that have a classic "dinner fork" deformity are called
       _____ fractures.

   a.    Volkmann's
   b.    Homan's
   c.    Colles'
   d.    Brown's

66.    Placing a roller bandage in the hand prior to splinting fractures places the hand
       in the position of:

   a.    extension
   b.    rotation
   c.    function
   d.    articulation

Match the splinting method in column B with the fracture or dislocation in column A.

| Column A | Column B |
|---|---|
| C 67.    dislocated shoulder | a.    traction splint |
| E 68.    fractured ankle | b.    rigid 3 foot and 5 foot splint |
| F 69.    fractured hand | |
| | c.    sling and swathe |
| B 70.    fractured tibia | |
| | d.    tongue blade splint |
| D 71.    fractured finger | |
| | e.    pillow splint |
| A 72.    fractured femur | |
| | f.    rigid 9 inch splint |

73. Instability of the pelvis suggests a minimum of ___ fractures of the pelvic ring.

     a. 2
     b. 3
     c. 4
     d. 5

74. The stability of the pelvis is evaluated by gentle compression of the iliac bones medially and:

     a. anteriorly
     b. laterally
     c. posteriorly
     d. superiorly

75. Multiple fractures of the pelvis associated with hypovolemic shock is best treated by application of:

     a. a traction splint
     b. PASG (MAST trousers)
     c. 3 and 5 foot rigid splint
     d. tying the legs together

76. By far, the most common hip dislocation is a(n) _____ dislocation.

     a. anterior
     b. posterior
     c. central
     d. lateral

Match the mechanism of injury in column B with the type of hip dislocation in column A.

| Column A | | Column B | |
|---|---|---|---|
| C 77. | anterior | a. | car dashboard against knee |
| A 78. | posterior | | |
| | | b. | lateral blow to hip |
| B 79. | central | | |
| | | c. | lateral rotational force to lower leg |

80. When the thigh is flexed, adducted and internally rotated, it is highly suggestive of a(n) _____ hip dislocation.

     a. anterior
     b. posterior
     c. central
     d. lateral

81.    When the thigh is flexed, abducted and externally rotated, it is highly suggestive
       of a(n) _____ hip dislocation.

       a.    anterior
       b.    posterior
       c.    central
       d.    lateral

82.    The classic presentation resulting from a hip fracture is:

       a.    internal rotation and shortening
       b.    internal rotation and thigh flexion
       c.    external rotation and shortening
       d.    external rotation and thigh flexion

Match the description in column B with the appropriate traction splint in column A.
One description can be used twice.

| Column A | | Column B | |
|---|---|---|---|
| B 83. | Hare | a. | single bar and pulley that can be placed either medial or lateral |
| B 84. | Kippel | | |
| A 85. | Sager | b. | double bar with ischial ring and strap, that is tightened with a pulley |

86.    The lower leg bone that can be palpated on the anterior lower leg is the:

       a.    fibula
       b.    radius
       c.    tibia
       d.    talus

87.    Which of the following fractures is commonly associated with spine injuries?

       a.    patella
       b.    calcaneus
       c.    metatarsal
       d.    hip

88.    Pelvic fractures in stable patients are best splinted by:

       a.    rigid 3 and 5 foot splints
       b.    securing patient to long spine board
       c.    traction splint application
       d.    PASG application

*Chapter 10*

## Case Histories

| Case History #1 |
|---|

You respond to a call and find 83 year old female patient complaining of pain in the mid-thigh region. She states that she fell from a ladder and landed on her foot and heel. However, the leg feels quite stable and she is able to walk on it.

89. Based on the history, what type of fracture might this patient most likely have sustained?

    a. an impacted femur fracture
    b. a comminuted femur fracture
    c. a dislocated hip
    d. a fractured hip

90. The mechanism of injury for this patient is best described as:

    a. direct
    b. twisting
    c. indirect
    d. rotational

91. The splint of choice for this patient is:

    a. traction
    b. pillow
    c. 3 inch lateral splints
    d. long spine board

| Case History #2 |
|---|

You find 6 year old boy who fell from a swing and landed on an outstretched hand. He complains of pain in his the mid portion of his lower arm. You note discoloration and swelling halfway between the wrist and the elbow, but the arm is stable.

92. Based on the age of the patient, history and physical exam, you suspect a _____ fracture.

    a. spiral
    b. greenstick
    c. pathologic
    d. stress

93. The bones that are most likely fractured include the ulna and:

    a.    carpal bones
    b.    humerus
    c.    olecranon
    d.    radius

94. The splint of choice for this patient is a sling and swathe with a:

    a.    pillow splint
    b.    18 inch rigid board splint
    c.    9 inch rigid board splint
    d.    Sager splint

---

### Case History #3

You respond to a call and find 24 year old ice skater who fell on an outstretched arm and is complaining of shoulder pain. She is supporting her forearm with her opposite hand, and her upper arm is positioned slightly away from her chest wall on the injured side. You note deformity and tenderness in the shoulder region.

---

95. Based on the history and physical exam, you suspect a(n):

    a.    fracture shaft of the humerus
    b.    anterior shoulder dislocation
    c.    fracture of the scapula
    d.    fracture of the olecranon

96. The splint of choice for this patient is a(n):

    a.    rigid board splint
    b.    air splint
    c.    pillow splint
    d.    sling and swathe

97. Given the site and nature of this injury, what complication are you most concerned about in this patient?

    a.    hemorrhage at the site of injury
    b.    fat embolism
    c.    neurovascular compromise
    d.    poor healing

---

### Case History #4

---

You respond to a call and find 74 year old male patient complaining of hip pain. He states that he simply stepped off a high curb and planted his foot forcefully on the ground and felt severe pain in his hip. He is lying on the ground, and his leg appears externally rotated and shortened.

---

98.  Based on the history and physical exam, you suspect a:

 a.  minor muscle injury
 b.  dislocation of the hip
 c.  fracture of the hip
 d.  pelvic fracture

99.  Given the minor nature of the mechanism of injury, what preexisting condition might explain this injury?

 a.  osteoporosis
 b.  arteriosclerosis
 c.  hypercalcemia
 d.  stress injury

100.  The splint of choice for this patient is:

 a.  traction splint
 b.  board splint
 c.  pillow splint
 d.  air splint

---

### Case History #5

---

A 45 year old construction worker fell from a 20 foot scaffold and landed on his feet. He is pale, sweaty and has delayed capillary refill. His blood pressure is 80/60, and his pulse is 140 and regular. You note that his left leg is deformed at the mid thigh region and at the mid lower leg. His right leg appears normal, but he has no dorsalis pedis or posterior tibial pulses in either leg.

---

101.  Based on the above history and physical exam, your immediate concern is:

 a.  loosing the extremities due to poor blood supply
 b.  decompensated hypovolemic shock
 c.  causing open fractures during transport
 d.  paralysis of the right leg

102. The absence of pulses in both legs is probably related to:

    a. the vasoconstriction response of shock
    b. compression of an artery due to fractures
    c. swelling in the thighs
    d. peripheral nerve injury

103. The treatment of choice for the fractures in this patient is:

    a. traction
    b. PASG
    c. board splints
    d. air splints

---

### Case History #6

A 40 year old female pedestrian is struck in the left knee region by an automobile. You note the leg is grossly angulated at the left knee, and pulses are absent on the injured side. The patient also has a "dinner fork" deformity in her right wrist. Otherwise the patient is stable and has no other obvious injuries.

---

104. Based on the above finding you should:

    a. splint the leg as you found it
    b. attempt gentle straightening to regain pulse
    c. apply traction with a Hare or Sager splint
    d. elevate the limb in the angulated position

105. The wrist injury best describes a _____ fracture.

    a. Volkmann
    b. Homan
    c. Colles'
    d. Brown

106. The hand and wrist should be placed in the position of function and splinted with a:

    a. traction splint
    b. rigid splint
    c. pillow splint
    d. sling and swathe

---

### Case History #7

You respond to a head-on automobile collision and find a 25 year old male complaining of pain in his chest, abdomen and left leg. His blood pressure is 70/50, and his pulse is 42 and regular. He is pale, cool and sweaty, and his lips are cyanotic. You note that his left leg is flexed at the hip, adducted and internally rotated.

---

107. Based on the above history and physical exam, your immediate actions would consist of:

    a. extricate rapidly, immobilize spine, administer oxygen and transport
    b. extricate with KED, immobilize leg and spine, administer oxygen and transport
    c. administer oxygen, perform secondary survey in car, splint leg, immobilize spine and transport
    d. administer oxygen, extricate with KED, splint leg, immobilize spine and transport

108. Based on the presentation of the leg you suspect a:

    a. fractured femur
    b. fractured hip
    c. dislocation of the hip
    d. fractured pelvis

Skill Performance Sheet

## Applying a Sling and Swathe

Student Name_____          Date_____

| Performance Standard | Performed | Failed |
|---|---|---|
| Support extremity during procedure | | |
| Expose and examines extremity | | |
| Check distal pulse and function | | |
| Place sling with long end over opposite shoulder and apex toward injured side | | |
| Tie sling at side of neck to avoid pressure | | |
| Secure end of sling with knot or twist | | |
| Attach swathes | | |
| Check distal pulse and function | | |
| Leave fingernails exposed | | |

Comments_____

_____

_____

_____

Instructor _____          Circle One:   Pass   Fail

Skill Performance Sheet

# Rigid Splinting for Humerus Fracture

Student Name_____          Date_____

| Performance Standard | Performed | Failed |
|---|---|---|
| Check distal pulse | | |
| Apply 9 inch splint to medial arm | | |
| Apply sling | | |
| Attach swathe | | |
| Check distal pulse and function | | |
| Leave fingernails exposed | | |

Comments_____

_____

_____

_____

Instructor _____          Circle One:   Pass   Fail

Skill Performance Sheet

# Splinting the Arm in the Straightened Position

Student Name_____          Date_____

| Performance Standard | Performed | Failed |
|---|---|---|
| Maintain immobilization distal and proximal to injury | | |
| Check distal pulse | | |
| Place splints medial and lateral | | |
| Attach splints with cravats or bandage | | |
| Attach arm to body with cravats | | |
| Check distal pulse and function | | |

Comments_____

_____

_____

_____

Instructor _____          Circle One:  Pass  Fail

Skill Performance Sheet

# Splinting the Elbow in an Angulated Position

Student Name_____          Date_____

| Performance Standard | Performed | Failed |
|---|---|---|
| Check distal pulse | | |
| Bridge splint from upper arm to forearm | | |
| Attach with cravats or bandage | | |
| Place sling without direct pressure on elbow | | |
| Check distal pulse and function | | |

Comments_____

_____

_____

_____

Instructor _____          Circle One:   Pass   Fail

Skill Performance Sheet

# Splinting the Wrist

Student Name_____     Date_____

| Performance Standard | Performed | Failed |
|---|---|---|
| Check capillary refill | | |
| Maintain distal and proximal immobilization, and position splint medially | | |
| Place hand in position of function with rolled bandage or gauze | | |
| Attach splint with cravats or bandage | | |
| Apply sling and swathe (optional) and elevate hand | | |
| Check distal circulation and function | | |

Comments_____

_____

_____

_____

Instructor _____     Circle One:   Pass   Fail

Skill Performance Sheet

# Applying a Finger Splint

Student Name_____          Date_____

| Performance Standard | Performed | Failed |
|---|---|---|
| Check capillary refill | | |
| Position finger splint or tongue blade from fingertip to heel of hand | | |
| Tape splint in place | | |
| Apply sling and elevate hand | | |
| Check distal circulation and function | | |

Comments_____

_____

_____

_____

Instructor _____          Circle One:   Pass   Fail

Skill Performance Sheet

## Applying an Air Splint

Student Name_____          Date_____

| Performance Standard | Performed | Failed |
|---|---|---|
| Check distal pulse | | |
| EMT #1 maintains distal and proximal immobilization | | |
| EMT #2 wraps splint on his or her arm | | |
| Slide splint onto patient's arm | | |
| Inflate splint | | |
| Check for correct pressure by pressing small dent in splint | | |
| Check distal pulse and function | | |

Comments_____

_____

_____

_____

Instructor _____          Circle One:   Pass   Fail

Skill Performance Sheet

# Applying a Hare Traction Splint

Student Name_____          Date_____

| Performance Standard | Performed | Failed |
|---|---|---|
| EMT #1 checks distal pulse while | | |
| EMT #2 maintains immobilization at the knee | | |
| Cut pants away | | |
| Inspect injured area | | |
| Attach ankle hitch and maintain traction with ankle hitch | | |
| Measure and adjust length of splint | | |
| Place splint with ischial bar at base of buttocks | | |
| Apply traction with crank until patient feels comfort or length of injured leg matches good leg | | |
| Attach straps above and below knee | | |
| Check distal pulse and function | | |

Comments_____

_____

_____

_____

Instructor _____          Circle One:  Pass  Fail

Skill Performance Sheet

## Applying a Sager Traction Splint

Student Name_____          Date_____

| Performance Standard | Performed | Failed |
|---|---|---|
| Check distal pulse | | |
| EMT #1 maintains immobilization at knee | | |
| Position splint and attach ischial strap | | |
| Attach the ankle hitch | | |
| Apply traction with ankle hitch by pulling bar | | |
| Apply supports over upper and lower leg | | |
| Check distal pulse and function | | |

Comments_____

_____

_____

_____

Instructor _____          Circle One:   Pass   Fail

Skill Performance Sheet

# Applying a Rigid Leg Splint

Student Name_____        Date_____

| Performance Standard | Performed | Failed |
|---|---|---|
| EMT #1 maintains immobilization | | |
| EMT #2 cuts away pants and checks distal pulse | | |
| Align splints on medial and lateral sides of the legs | | |
| Attach splints with cravats or bandages | | |
| Elevate leg | | |
| Check distal pulse and function | | |

Comments_____

_____

_____

_____

Instructor _____        Circle One:   Pass   Fail

Skill Performance Sheet

# Applying a Pillow Splint to the Ankle

Student Name_____        Date_____

| Performance Standard | Performed | Failed |
|---|---|---|
| Check distal pulse | | |
| Wrap pillow around heel and ankle | | |
| Attach with cravats or bandages | | |
| Check distal circulation and function | | |

Comments_____

_____

_____

_____

Instructor _____        Circle One:   Pass   Fail

## Chapter 11

## ENVIRONMENTAL EMERGENCIES

1.    Heat production in the body is primarily a function of the:

   a.   metabolism
   b.   skin
   c.   gastrointestinal tract
   d.   kidneys

2.    The transfer of heat from a warmer to a cooler environment not in direct contact with the body is called:

   a.   evaporation
   b.   conduction
   c.   convection
   d.   radiation

3.    The transfer of heat to objects in direct contact with the body is called:

   a.   evaporation
   b.   conduction
   c.   convection
   d.   radiation

4.    The transfer of heat to circulating air currents is called:

   a.   evaporation
   b.   conduction
   c.   convection
   d.   radiation

5.    The loss of heat when moisture vaporizes on the body surface is called:

   a.   evaporation
   b.   conduction
   c.   convection
   d.   radiation

6.    Under normal conditions, most heat loss occurs via:

   a.   evaporation
   b.   conduction
   c.   convection
   d.   radiation

7.     Loss of heat via respiration is:

    a.     large
    b.     moderate
    c.     minimal
    d.     not possible

8.     The body's "thermostat" that regulates temperature by influencing heat production, heat distribution and heat loss is located in the:

    a.     cerebellum
    b.     brainstem
    c.     hypothalmus
    d.     pituitary

9.     Heat distribution and heat loss are a primary responsibility of the:

    a.     cardiovascular system
    b.     respiratory system
    c.     digestive system
    d.     urinary system

10.    When heat loss is needed, the body responds by initiating _____ in the skin.

    a.     vasoconstriction
    b.     vasodilation
    c.     shivering
    d.     piloerection

11.    High humidity in the environment will decrease the rate of _____ since the air is already saturated with water.

    a.     convection
    b.     conduction
    c.     respiration
    d.     evaporation

12.    Excessive losses of salt during exercise can cause heat:

    a.     exhaustion
    b.     cramps
    c.     prostration
    d.     stroke

13. To ensure a balanced intake of water and electrolytes, drinks such as
    _____ are effective.

    a. sugar water
    b. Gatorade
    c. orange juice
    d. seltzer

14. Which of the following age groups are most susceptible to heat emergencies?

    a. teenagers
    b. elderly
    c. middle aged
    d. none of the above

Match the explanations in column B to the predisposing factors of heat-related
emergencies in column A.

| Column A | Column B |
|---|---|
| A 15. heart disease | a. compromised cardiovascular response |
| B 16. obesity | b. increased insulation results in less heat loss |
| C 17. febrile illness | |
| D 18. Parkinson's disease | c. increased heat production |
| E 19. mental retardation | d. muscle tremors produce heat |
| | e. inability to care for themselves |

20. Alcohol causes _____ and can cause a gain in heat when the
    environmental temperature is above body temperature.

    a. vasoconstriction
    b. vasodilation
    c. increased pulse
    d. high blood pressure

21. Muscle cramping in heavily used muscles either during or immediately
    following exertion best describes:

    a. heat exhaustion
    b. heat stroke
    c. heat prostration
    d. heat cramps

22. The problem in the previous question should be treated by all of the following <u>except</u>:

    a. rapid cooling with ice water
    b. placing the patient in a cool location
    c. providing an electrolyte drink
    d. stretching crampy muscles

23. The heat disorder that results from widespread vasodilation and fluid loss from sweating is called:

    a. heat exhaustion
    b. heat stroke
    c. heat prostration
    d. heat cramps

24. The treatment of the above condition includes all of the following <u>except</u>:

    a. rapid cooling with ice water
    b. removal to cool environment
    c. removal excessive clothing
    d. replacement of electrolyte fluids

Match the signs and symptoms in column B with the heat-related condition in column A.

| Column A | Column B |
|---|---|
| C 25. heat exhaustion | a. very high temperature, dry skin and altered mental state |
| B 26. heat cramps | b. muscular cramps following exercise |
| A 27. heat stroke | c. weakness, cool sweaty skin, rapid pulse and elevated core temperature |

D 28. The treatment of heat stroke involves all of the following <u>except</u>:

    a. rapid cooling with ice at arterial points
    b. fanning with wet sheets on body
    c. rapid transport and oxygen
    d. cooling with alcohol sponge bath

29.    On a hot, dry and windless day (99° F), the body relies primarily on which of the following mechanisms to loose heat?

       a.    convection
       b.    evaporation
       c.    radiation
       d.    respiration

30.    A core body temperature of less than 35°C best defines:

       a.    frostbite
       b.    chillblains
       c.    hypothermia
       d.    frostnip

31.    A normal body response to cold emergencies involves:

       a.    increased metabolism and vasoconstriction at skin
       b.    increased metabolism and vasodilation at skin
       c.    slowed metabolism and vasoconstriction at skin
       d.    slowed metabolism and vasodilation at skin

32.    Acute immersion hypothermia is a very severe form of cold injury because:

       a.    water is a very good conductor of heat
       b.    water vapors freeze your nasal mucosa
       c.    inhalation of water causes bronchoconstriction
       d.    cold water causes vasodilation and shock

33.    A person who is drug intoxicated, ill and lying on the floor of their apartment (70°F) for 2 days becomes hypothermic.  This is an example of:

       a.    subacute hypothermia
       b.    acute hypothermia
       c.    chronic hypothermia
       d.    chillblains

## Chapter 11

Categorize the items in column A as either mild, moderate or severe signs or symptoms of hypothermia.

| Column A | | Column B | |
|---|---|---|---|
| C 34. | significant hypotension | a. | mild (35°-33°C) |
| C 35. | unresponsive to pain | b. | moderate (32°-27°C) |
| A 36. | difficulty in speech | c. | severe (26°-22°C) |
| B 37. | muscular rigidity | | |
| B 38. | slowing of pulse and respirations | | |
| C 39. | ventricular fibrillation | | |
| A 40. | shivering | | |

41. Which of the following statements regarding active external rewarming (i.e., placing the patient in a tub with 105°F water) is most correct?

    a. it is essential for all patients to avoid brain damage
    b. it should only be for severe hypothermia when pulse rate is less than 50
    c. it should only be used when transport is significantly delayed or after acute immersion
    d. it should never be used

42. Which of the following statements regarding stimulation of hypothermic patients is most correct?

    a. they should receive vigorous tactile stimulation so that they do not lapse into coma
    b. they should be handled very gently to avoid abnormal heart rhythms
    c. they should receive strong verbal stimulation to increase circulation to the brain
    d. they should receive only vigorous stimulation when they are in coma

43. With severe hypothermia patients, hyperventilation should be:

    a. avoided
    b. performed at 24 breaths\min
    c. performed at 32 breaths\min
    d. performed at 40 breaths\min

44.  Which of the active rewarming techniques is recommended for field use?

   a.  gastric lavage with warm fluids through a nasogastric tube
   b.  warm IV fluids and peritoneal lavage
   c.  warmed humidified oxygen and warm packs at arterial points (i.e., armpits)
   d.  applying battery-operated heated electric blankets

45.  CPR should be started on hypothermic patients when:

   a.  the pulse drops below 50
   b.  the pulse drops below 40
   c.  the pulse drops below 30
   d.  pulselessness is absolutely certain

46.  A major complication of active external rewarming is:

   a.  burns to the skin
   b.  respiratory arrest due to brainstem stimulation
   c.  rewarming shock due to vasodilation of peripheral vessels
   d.  damage to the respiratory mucosa

47.  Which of the following areas of the body is most subject to localized cold injury?

   a.  nose
   b.  genitalia
   c.  legs
   d.  arms

48.  Ironically, which of the following mechanisms that protect against hypothermia is the major contributor to localized cold injury?

   a.  increased heart rate
   b.  peripheral vasoconstriction
   c.  shivering
   d.  peripheral vasodilation

49.  A completely reversible cold injury characterized by blanching of the skin and loss of sensation in the affected area is called:

   a.  frostbite
   b.  chillblains
   c.  frostnip
   d.  superficial frostbite

50. A localized cold injury that is characterized by white and waxy skin that is firm to the touch but in which the tissue beneath the skin is soft and resilient is called:

    a. deep frostbite
    b. focal hypothermia
    c. frostnip
    d. superficial frostbite

51. The most severe form of localized cold injury that appears white and feels deeply frozen and resists depression to the touch is called:

    a. deep frostbite
    b. focal hypothermia
    c. frostnip
    d. superficial frostbite

52. Active rewarming of a frostbitten extremity is not recommended in the field because:

    a. of the time needed to effectively rewarm the part
    b. arrythmias may develop
    c. it can lead to rewarming shock
    d. it is performed with electrical equipment

53. If a frostbitten foot should thaw prior to arrival at the hospital, you should:

    a. break blisters to relieve pressure
    b. cover with sterile dressings
    c. encourage the person to walk to improve circulation
    d. do nothing to the affected part

54. In a wilderness situation in which transport is not possible, rewarming of a localized cold injury should be performed at water temperatures of:

    a. 100°F
    b. 102°F
    c. 105°F
    d. 110°F

55.    During the active rewarming process, water should:

   a.    remain perfectly still in the container to avoid irritation to the affected part
   b.    be continuously circulated to maintain an even temperature
   c.    be allowed to cool to body temperature during the rewarming process
   d.    be continuously heated slowly up to the patient's tolerance (not to exceed 120°F)

56.    Following the rewarming of a deeply frostbitten extremity, pain is:

   a.    common
   b.    very rare
   c.    occasional
   d.    highly unlikely

57.    Prolonged exposure (10-12 hours) to above-freezing temperatures and dampness (generally below 10°C, 50°F) can result in cold injury to wet extremities which is called:

   a.    chillblains
   b.    immersion foot
   c.    frostfoot
   d.    cold foot

58.    An abnormal vascular response to mild cold that manifests as itching, redness and swelling on the dorsal surfaces of the hands and feet following exposure to above-freezing temperatures is called:

   a.    chillblains
   b.    hyperemia
   c.    hypothermia dermatitis
   d.    puritus

59.    The two most critical variables in thermal burn injuries are:

   a.    degree of heat and length of exposure
   b.    type of heat and thickness of skin
   c.    distance from patient and pigment of skin
   d.    age of patient and pigment of skin

60.    Skin that is blistered, red and blotchy, and swollen and very painful best describes a ___ degree burn.

   a.    first
   b.    second
   c.    third
   d.    fourth

61. Which layer is injured in a first degree burn?

    a.    the dermis
    b.    the subcutaneous
    c.    the epidermis
    d.    the fascia

62. Damage to bone from a thermal injury suggests a minimum of a _____ degree burn.

    a.    second
    b.    third
    c.    fourth
    d.    fifth

63. The most common cause of a first degree burn is:

    a.    scalding injury
    b.    sunburn
    c.    electrical injury
    d.    chemical injury

64. Which of the following burn types is likely to be most painful?

    a.    first degree
    b.    second degree
    c.    third degree
    d.    fourth degree

65. Skin that appears charred, yellow brown, dark red, or white and translucent with thrombosed veins that are visible is probably related to a(n) _____ degree burn.

    a.    first
    b.    second
    c.    third
    d.    either first or second

66. A major complication of circumferential burns (completely around a body part such as the arm) is that they can:

    a.    increase lactic acid production
    b.    obstruct blood flow to the part
    c.    increase heat to the cells beneath
    d.    kill all superficial nerves

Match the burned body parts in column B to the correct percentage in column A.

| Column A | | Column B | |
|---|---|---|---|
| B 67. | 27% | a. | a baby's entire head |
| C 68. | 36% | b. | one leg and one arm of an adult |
| A 69. | 18% | c. | both arms and the anterior surface of both legs in an adult |
| D 70. | 9% | | |
| E 71. | 46% | d. | an adult's entire head |
| F 72. | 50% | e. | both legs, the groin and one arm of an adult |
| | | f. | the entire anterior surface of an adult |

73. Which of the following body areas is considered critical when evaluating a burn patient?

   a. armpits
   b. scalp
   c. perineum
   d. thigh

74. Charring around the mouth and nose, black sputum and singed nasal hairs and eyebrows are considered critical signs of:

   a. respiratory burn injuries
   b. eye injuries
   c. chemical burn injuries
   d. electrical injuries

75. All of the following are considered complicating factors in burn patients except:

   a. lighter skin pigment
   b. elderly patients
   c. preexisting cardiac and pulmonary disease
   d. small children

List the following burn management steps in chronological order by assigning the numbers 1 through 5 to the treatment steps.

5 76.   apply sterile dressing

3 77.   administer high concentration oxygen

2 78.   open the airway

4 79.   remove rings and bracelets

1 80.   stop the burning process

81.   The best dressing for a thermal burn is:

 a.   petroleum gauze
 b.   dry sterile wrap
 c.   plastic wrap
 d.   moist sterile

82.   A <u>common</u> major complication of large surface area burns is:

 a.   cardiac arrhythmias
 b.   hypothermia
 c.   pulmonary embolus
 d.   bone infections

83.   The most common cause of death from fires is:

 a.   fluid loss
 b.   infection
 c.   airway obstruction
 d.   smoke inhalation

84.   The most common toxic gas that is inhaled in a fire is:

 a.   phosgene
 b.   carbon dioxide
 c.   carbon monoxide
 d.   cyanide

85.   A early complication of direct heat transfer and burns to the respiratory tract is:

 a.   pulmonary fibrosis
 b.   bronchitis secondary to mucus production
 c.   airway obstruction
 d.   pulmonary embolus

86. Carbon monoxide is a particularly toxic gas since it has a 200 times greater affinity for _____ than does oxygen.

    a. diffusion
    b. inhalation
    c. hemoglobin
    d. cell bonding

87. Smoke inhalation patients with a cherry red color have probably achieved toxic levels of _____ inhalation.

    a. phosgene
    b. carbon dioxide
    c. carbon monoxide
    d. cyanide

88. Stridor and hoarseness may suggest _____ in burn patients:

    a. bronchiole injury
    b. alveoli irritation
    c. airway obstruction
    d. nasal burns

89. In general, the most effective treatment for chemical burn injuries is:

    a. application of cold packs on the affected area
    b. irrigation with copious amounts of water
    c. application of sterile dressing
    d. application of gels to smother burning process

90. Treatment of alkali burns requires:

    a. application of a neutralizing agent
    b. irrigation for 20-30 minutes
    c. submersion in a small tub of water
    d. rapid transport only

Match the <u>specific</u> treatments that are needed (either in the emergency department or in the industrial setting) in column B to the agent in column A.

| Column A | Column B |
|---|---|
| D 91. dried lime | a. submersion in water |
| A 92. phosphorus | b. application of calcium gluconate dressing |
| C 93. sodium and potassium metals | |
| B 94. hydrofluoric acid | c. coverage with petroleum jelly |
| E 95. phenols | d. brushing off before irrigation |
| | e. irrigation with 2:1 mixture of polyethylene glycol and mentholated spirits |

96.  The force with which the movement of electrical current occurs is:

    a.    amperage
    b.    voltage
    c.    resistance
    d.    wattage

97.  The number or volume of flowing electrons is called:

    a.    amperage
    b.    voltage
    c.    resistance
    d.    wattage

98.  The degree of hindrance to electron flow is called:

    a.    amperage
    b.    voltage
    c.    resistance
    d.    wattage

99.  Generally speaking, voltage:

    a.    causes more injury as it increases
    b.    causes less injury as it increases
    c.    does not affect the degree of injury
    d.    cannot cause death when less than 60 cycles per second

100. If electrical current passes through the brain, the primary complication is most likely to be:

    a. cardiac arrest
    b. cardiac arrhythmias
    c. respiratory arrest
    d. coronary thrombosis

101. Which of the following materials provides the greatest degree of resistance to electrical flow?

    a. water
    b. rubber
    c. copper
    d. steel

102. A large conducting body, such as the earth, that is used as a common return for an electrical circuit and an arbitrary zero of potential best describes:

    a. current
    b. voltage
    c. flow
    d. ground

103. The best action to take when a downed power line is in contact with the car you occupy is to:

    a. step out of the car quickly
    b. step out of the car if you have rubber soles
    c. stay in the car until power experts arrive
    d. step out of the car slowly

104. Wet skin offers _____ resistance to electricity.

    a. low
    b. high
    c. very high
    d. no

105. High voltage traveling through air and generating intense heat that can cause thermal burns is called a(n) _____ burn.

    a. air
    b. jump
    c. light
    d. arc

106. Which of the following is a complication of electrical current flowing through skeletal muscle?

    a.     fat tumors due to the release of lipoproteins
    b.     hyperglycemia due to glucagon release
    c.     contractions preventing release of a grasped electrical source
    d.     explosion of the muscle and skin

107. The process of emitting radiant energy, specifically the energy of electromagnetic waves in the form of waves or particles, best defines:

    a.     heat
    b.     radiation
    c.     contamination
    d.     isotope

108. Any radiation that displaces electrons from atoms or molecules and thereby produces ions, best defines:

    a.     roentgen
    b.     ionizing radiation
    c.     contamination
    d.     rem

109. The ability of a substance to emit rays or particles from its nucleus best defines:

    a.     radiowaves
    b.     radioactive
    c.     curie
    d.     isotope

110. The process by which radioactive material is removed from a person or object is called:

    a.     sweeping
    b.     decontamination
    c.     isotope brushing
    d.     deionization

111. All of the following are possibles sources of radiation accidents, <u>except</u>:

    a.     transportation accident
    b.     industrial setting
    c.     hospital
    d.     microwave oven

112. A term used to describe someone who is exposed to ionizing radiation but not contaminated is:

    a. irradiated
    b. absorbed
    c. factored
    d. quantified

113. The smallest building block of an element is a(n):

    a. cell
    b. micron
    c. atom
    d. tissue

Match the type of radiation in column B to the description in column A.

| Column A | | Column B | |
|---|---|---|---|
| A 114. | the least penetrating form of radiation and that travels only a few centimeters in the air | a. | alpha |
| | | b. | gamma |
| B 115. | high energy electromagnetic radiation similar to x-rays; can penetrate and cause severe damage to tissues, but cannot contaminate others in contact with the patient | c. | beta |
| C 116. | can travel 1 foot to several feet and can penetrate into the dermal layer of the skin; can contaminate the patient and make him or her a danger to others | | |

117. A patient who has radioactive particles on his or her body and is a danger to others is said to be:

    a. irradiated
    b. active
    c. contaminated
    d. ionized

118. A patient who has inhaled or swallowed solid radioactive materials is an example of:

    a. internal contamination
    b. external contamination
    c. irradiation
    d. activation

119.  A radiation monitoring instrument that records the total accumulated dose of radiation is called a:

    a.    survey instrument
    b.    dosimeter
    c.    Geiger counter
    d.    radioisotope

120.  A radiation monitoring instrument that monitors the rate of exposure in roentgens or milliroentgens per hour is called a:

    a.    survey instrument
    b.    dosimeter
    c.    Geiger-Mueller counter
    d.    a and c

121.  All of the following are factors that affect the severity of a radiation exposure except:

    a.    type of radiation
    b.    the temperature in the area
    c.    area of the body exposed
    d.    distance from the source

122.  All of the following are sources of information at the site of a potential transportation radiation accident except:

    a.    shipping papers
    b.    the color of the vehicle
    c.    placards on the vehicle
    d.    the driver of the vehicle

123.  A national organization that can be consulted in the event of a radiation for information on how to proceed goes by which of the following initials?

    a.    AHA
    b.    REAC/TS
    c.    NACOT
    d.    RADS

124.  In the event that you are part of a rescue team who must enter an area of potential radiation exposure (i.e., a Chernobyl-like circumstance), which of the following persons is least suited for the rescue according to the national council on radiation protection and measurements?

    a.    a 20 year old female volunteer firefighter
    b.    a 50 year old male volunteer firefighter
    c.    a 25 year old male volunteer firefighter
    d.    a 50 year old women volunteer firefighter

125. The DOT emergency response guidebook recommends a safety zone at a radiation accident be <u>at least</u> _____ feet upwind from the accident.

    a. 50
    b. 100
    c. 150
    d. 500

126. When working with patients at a radiation accident, the <u>absolute minimum</u> of protective clothing should include:

    a. gloves and goggles
    b. gloves, mask, gown and shoe covers
    c. goggles and gown
    d. scuba gear, gown, rubber boots

127. Prior to bringing a contaminated patient into the emergency department, you should:

    a. identify the correct designated "dirty" path and room to bring the patient to
    b. remove all blankets from the patients and carry them into the emergency department
    c. remove your protective clothing and bring the patient to the room
    d. hand carry all contaminated material in before you bring the patient into the emergency room

128. Upon arrival in the emergency department you should remove your contaminated clothing in what order?

    a. outer gloves, tape at sleeves and cuffs, surgical gown and shirt, head cover, shoe cover, inner gloves
    b. outer gloves, inner gloves, shoe cover, tape at sleeves and cuffs, surgical gown and shirt, head cover
    c. tape at sleeves and cuffs, surgical gown and shirt, head cover, shoe cover, outer gloves, inner gloves
    d. surgical gown, outer gloves, tape at sleeves and cuffs, gown and shirt, head cover, shoe cover, inner gloves

129. As one descends in water or from high altitudes, the pressure becomes:

    a. less
    b. more
    c. more in air and less in water
    d. more in water and less in air

130. When a diver ascends too rapidly (faster than 60 feet/min) nitrogen bubbles can form in tissues and the bloodstream, resulting in a condition called decompression sickness, Caisson's disease or:

    a. barotrauma
    b. altitude sickness
    c. hydroencephalopathy
    d. the bends

131. All of the following are a possible signs and symptoms of decompression sickness <u>except</u>:

    a. vomiting blood
    b. difficulty breathing
    c. alteration of consciousness
    d. vertigo or spinning sensation

132. The deep and burning pain of decompression sickness is most often felt in the _____ since this area can least tolerate the expansion of tissues.

    a. mid thigh
    b. joints
    c. head
    d. chest

133. A patient who is suspected of having decompression sickness should be placed _____ with head and chest inclined downward to prevent air bubbles from entering the heart.

    a. supine
    b. prone
    c. on the left side
    d. on the right side

134. The definitive treatment for decompression sickness is:

    a. surgical removal of nitrogen bubbles
    b. treatment in a hyperbaric chamber
    c. rapid infusion of air-dissolving drugs
    d. observation and free-flow oxygen therapy

135. Injury to body cavities during changes in altitude due to unequal pressures is called:

    a. barotrauma
    b. altitude sickness
    c. hydroencephalopathy
    d. the bends

136.    The <u>primary</u> responsibility of an EMT at a hazardous material incident is:

     a.     containment
     b.     decontamination
     c.     emergency medical care
     d.     removal

137.    You smell a strange odor when approaching a transportation accident; you should first:

     a.     relocate upwind and access the scene from a distance
     b.     apply your scuba gear and approach the scene to perform an assessment
     c.     move away from the scene until you cannot smell the substance and then perform an assessment
     d.     contact Chemtrec immediately to have an expert come to the scene

138.    When reacting to a documented HAZMAT incident, it is important to establish a patient treatment and transport location called a:

     a.     command center
     b.     staging area
     c.     communications area
     d.     triage area

139.    The bill of lading is most often found:

     a.     in the cab of the vehicle or with the driver
     b.     posted on the back end of the vehicle
     c.     posted on the side of the vehicle
     d.     posted on the front of the vehicle

## Case Histories

---

### Case History #1

A 78 year old man is found on a park bench on a hot and humid summer day. He is unresponsive to painful stimulus. The physical exam reveals hot, flushed, dry skin, and strong bounding pulse. His vital signs are respirations 28 and shallow, pulse 120 and regular, and blood pressure 190/110.

---

140.    This patient is probably suffering from:

     a.     a severe infection
     b.     heat stroke
     c.     heat exhaustion
     d.     heat cramps

141. The <u>primary</u> reason for the extremely hot temperature in this patient is failure of the _____ to help cool the patient.

    a. sweating mechanism
    b. vasodilation mechanism
    c. heart rate
    d. metabolism

142. The primary treatment needed to save this patient is:

    a. rapid cooling with alcohol soaks
    b. rapid cooling with water and convection
    c. gradual cooling in shade and with salt water drinks
    d. rapid transport only

---

### Case History #2

You respond to a marathon race and find a 23 year old male patient who collapsed in the 21st mile of the race on a very hot (98°F) and dry day. According to bystanders he fainted 10 minutes earlier and regained consciousness 1 minute before your arrival. Physical exam reveals the patient is lethargic and has pale and sweaty skin that is cool to the touch, weakness, dizziness and a headache. His vital signs are pulse 90 and regular, respirations 20 and shallow, and blood pressure 120/80. However, the blood pressure drops to 90/70 when the patient sits up.

---

143. This patient is probably suffering from:

    a. cardiac syncope
    b. heat stroke
    c. heat exhaustion
    d. heat cramps

144. Of the following, the <u>primary</u> reason for the fainting episode and the drop in blood pressure when sitting up is:

    a. loss of sodium
    b. widespread vasodilation
    c. the heart rate
    d. muscle weakness

145. The primary treatment needed to stabilize this patient is:

    a. rapid cooling with alcohol soaks
    b. rapid cooling with water and convection
    c. gradual cooling in shade and replacement of fluids
    d. rapid transport only

---

**Case History #3**

You respond to a school yard on a very hot and humid day and find a 16 year old girl complaining of severe leg cramps and sweating profusely . Otherwise, her physical exam and vital signs are normal. The coach advises you that she was running just prior to the episode.

---

146. This patient is probably suffering from:

   a. cardiac syncope
   b. simple muscle cramps
   c. heat exhaustion
   d. heat cramps

147. The <u>primary</u> reason for the cramping is:

   a. excessive loss of body salt
   b. widespread vasodilation
   c. muscle injury
   d. muscle weakness

148. The primary treatment needed to stabilize this patient is:

   a. rapid cooling with alcohol soaks
   b. rapid cooling with water and convection
   c. gradual cooling in shade and fluids
   d. rapid transport only

---

**Case History #4**

You respond to an apartment and find a 78 year old man who fell approximately 2 days ago and was found by his son 30 minutes before your arrival. The room is about 65°F. Physical exam reveals the patient is responsive to painful but not verbal stimuli, his skin is cool and dry to the touch, and he is shivering very slightly. His right leg is externally rotated and shortened, and his vital signs are pulse 80 and irregular, respirations 10 and shallow, and blood pressure 90/60. (The questions that follow include a partial review of Chapter 10.)

---

149. Based on the presentation of the leg this patient has probably:

   a. dislocated his right hip posteriorly
   b. fractured his right hip
   c. fractured the right side of his pelvis
   d. fractured his right knee

150. Of the following, the best explanation for this patient's mental state and vital signs is:

    a. cardiogenic shock
    b. shock due to pain in leg
    c. cardiac arrhythmia
    d. moderate hypothermia

151. The primary treatment needed to stabilize this patient is:

    a. warming with blankets
    b. hot drinks enroute to the hospital
    c. rapid warming with electric blankets
    d. rapid transport only

---

### Case History #5

You respond to a chemical manufacturing plant and find a 42 year old woman who has received an entire body splash with an acid solution. She is alert and oriented and is in severe pain.

---

152. Your immediate action should be to:

    a. provide rapid transport while irrigating with an IV solution enroute
    b. have the patient remove all of her clothing and place her in a shower to irrigate
    c. rinse the patient with an alkali solution to neutralize the acid
    d. irrigate with a mild acid solution (i.e., orange juice) to avoid a chemical reaction

153. This patient's skin should be irrigated for a minimum of:

    a. 3-5 minutes
    b. 5-10 minutes
    c. 10-15 minutes
    d. 15-20 minutes

154. If this substance was a dried chemical, what actions would you take before irrigating?

    a. neutralizing
    b. brushing off skin
    c. blowing off skin
    d. rubbing off skin

---

### Case History #6

---

A 42 year old man fell asleep while smoking in his den. His easy chair caught fire, and soon the house was in flames. The firemen bring the man out of the burning house to your ambulance. The patient has blistering burns on his head and entire neck (completely around), his anterior chest and abdomen, and his groin. He has singed nasal hairs and eyebrows, and there is soot within the nostrils. His voice is very hoarse, and he is exhibiting stridor. He is alert, and his vital signs are respirations 20 and regular, pulse 100 and regular, and blood pressure 140/70.

---

155.  What percentage of his body do you estimate is burned?

    a.    15%
    b.    21%
    c.    28%
    d.    35%

156.  The burned areas are probably:

    a.    first degree
    b.    second degree
    c.    third degree
    d.    fourth degree

157.  Based on your finding, how would you classify this burn using the American College of Surgeons criteria?

    a.    minor
    b.    moderate
    c.    major
    d.    minor to moderate

158.  What is your greatest concern regarding this patient?

    a.    hypovolemic shock due to fluid loss
    b.    airway obstruction due to respiratory burns
    c.    massive infection due to surface area
    d.    neurogenic distributive shock due to pain

159.  How should oxygen be provided?

    a.    via nasal cannula
    b.    humidified via nonrebreather mask
    c.    via bag-valve-mask
    d.    via manually triggered resuscitator mask

---

### Case History #7

You respond to a call and find a 2 year old boy who has bitten into an electrical wire and appears to be having a grand mal seizure. His father is in a panic and is unable to provide a history of what happened. The child appears to still be biting the wire.

---

160. The child is probably still in contact with the wire because:

    a. he is having tetanic contractions of his jaw
    b. the wire has adhered to the mucosa
    c. he has aspirated the wire into his pharynx
    d. the wire has looped around his teeth

161. Your immediate action would be to:

    a. call the power company to disconnect the electricity
    b. find the fuse box and disconnect the fuse
    c. pull the plug from the outlet
    d. hit the child with a piece of wood to disconnect him from the wire

162. Of the following, which offers the least resistance to electricity?

    a. muscles
    b. nerves
    c. bone
    d. fatty tissue

163. Once the child was disconnected from the wire, your first concern should be:

    a. severe internal burns
    b. destruction of the skeletal muscles
    c. respiratory status
    d. eye injuries due to burns

164. Given the location and nature of the event, you would also be concerned about:

    a. fracture or dislocation of the cervical vertebrae
    b. accessory muscle tears
    c. pneumothorax
    d. cardiac contusion

---

Case History #8

You find a 80 year old homeless man in an alley on a cold and windy day. You note that his hands are white and very cold to the touch. They feel firm on the superficial and deep layers of soft tissue.

---

165. Based on the description you suspect:

    a.    frostnip
    b.    superficial frostbite
    c.    deep frostbite
    d.    chillblains

166. You are 10 minutes from the hospital. Which of the following actions is <u>not</u> appropriate?

    a.    submerge in 105°F water during transport
    b.    insulate hands with loose material and transport
    c.    administer oxygen via face mask
    d.    remove wet clothing from the patient

---

Case History #9

You respond to a truck accident, and the police advise you that a carton containing beta radiation liquid material has been breached. The material has come in contact with the driver's hands. Upon examination you note no wounds on the hands.

---

167. You would describe this patient as:

    a.    irradiated
    b.    externally contaminated
    c.    internally contaminated
    d.    having absorbed radiation

168. The patient is a potential threat to:

    a.    only himself
    b.    anyone who comes in direct contact with him
    c.    anyone who comes within several yards
    d.    no one including himself

169. The radiological expert may issue you a _____ to measure your <u>accumulated dose</u> of radiation.

    a.    survey meter
    b.    Gieger counter
    c.    dosimeter
    d.    radiological monitor

---

### Case History #10

You find a 20 year old complaining of difficulty breathing and severe joint and ear pain. His friend states that he panicked during a dive about 1 hour ago and rapidly ascended from 150 feet.

---

170.  This patient's major problem is probably:

    a.    barotrauma
    b.    decompression sickness
    c.    pneumothorax
    d.    cardiac failure

171.  Rapid ascent can lead:

    a.    formation of gas bubbles in tissues and blood
    b.    swimmers ear
    c.    oxygen narcosis
    d.    diver's delusions

172.  The most important prehospital treatment for this patient is:

    a.    administering of 100% oxygen
    b.    elevating his head to avoid embolism
    c.    keeping him cool to prevent nitrogen absorption
    d.    resubmerging him to decompress

173.  Definitive treatment of this patient requires:

    a.    surgery
    b.    hyperbaric treatment
    c.    open heart massage
    d.    removing air bubble with IV therapy

## Chapter 12

## MEDICAL EMERGENCIES

1.  Diabetes is a disease that results from an inadequate secretion of the hormone:

    a.  insulin
    b.  epinephrine
    c.  glucagon
    d.  progesterone

2.  Insulin helps regulate the utilization and storage of:

    a.  ketones
    b.  isotones
    c.  glucose
    d.  epinephrine

3.  While most cells also use other sources of fuel, such as fats, the central nervous system depends almost exclusively on:

    a.  insulin
    b.  glycogen
    c.  glucose
    d.  glucagon

4.  Insulin is produced within specialized cells in the _____ called the islets of Langerhans.

    a.  liver
    b.  spleen
    c.  pancreas
    d.  adrenal gland

5.  Some glucose is stored in the liver and muscle as a larger molecule called:

    a.  glucagon
    b.  glycogen
    c.  fructose
    d.  insulin

6.  Many organs can burn fats for energy needs, but the _____ rely(ies) almost entirely primarily on glucose.

    a.  heart
    b.  lungs
    c.  kidneys
    d.  brain

7.    Stored forms of glucose can be released between meals.  This process is
      initiated by the hormone:

      a.    LDH
      b.    progesterone
      c.    glycogen
      d.    glucagon

8.    Patients who have a severe or absolute lack of insulin are called type ___, or
      insulin-dependent, diabetics.

      a.    I
      b.    II
      c.    III
      d.    IV

9.    Since the disease often develops early in life, type I diabetes is sometimes
      called _____ diabetes.

      a.    infantile
      b.    childhood
      c.    teenage
      d.    juvenile

10.   Type I diabetics require treatment with injections of:

      a.    glucose
      b.    glycogen
      c.    orinase
      d.    insulin

11.   Diabetic patients who usually develop diabetes later in life and may not
      require insulin injections are called non-insulin-dependent, or
      type_____, diabetics.

      a.    I
      b.    II
      c.    III
      d.    IV

12.   Non-insulin-dependent diabetics usually take medication that stimulates the
      pancreas to produce:

      a.    glucose
      b.    fructose
      c.    glycogen
      d.    insulin

13. Which of the following is a complication of diabetes?

    a. chronic lung disease
    b. atherosclerosis
    c. cancer
    d. Lou Gehrig's disease

14. A diabetic emergency that develops from a lack of insulin and elevated blood glucose causing dehydration and acidosis is:

    a. diabetic encephalopathy
    b. diabetic ketoacidosis
    c. diabetic syndrome
    d. insulin shock

Match the type of diabetic emergency in column B with the signs and symptoms in column A. Column B items can be used more than once.

| Column A | Column B |
| --- | --- |
| B 15. increased thirst | a. hypoglycemia |
| A 16 sweaty skin | b. diabetic ketoacidosis |
| A 17. pale skin | |
| B 18. increased urination | |
| B 19. abdominal pain (especially in children) | |
| A 20. combative behavior | |
| B 21. Kussmal's respiration | |
| B 22. fruity breath odor | |

23. The most common and treatable diabetic problem encountered in prehospital care that results from a lack of available sugar in the blood is:

    a. diabetic coma
    b. hypoglycemia
    c. hyperosmolar coma
    d. diabetic encephalopathy

24. The majority of signs and symptoms of hypoglycemia are related to:

    a. dehydration
    d. brain irritation
    c. acidosis
    d. signs of adrenaline release

25. Signs of hypoglycemia may include hunger, nausea, weakness and:

    a. dry mouth
    b. bizzare behavior
    c. slow pulse
    d. hypotension

26. A drug that is given intramuscularly for hypoglycemia and that may be carried at times by the patient is:

    a. glucose
    b. glucagon
    c. glycogen
    d. insulin

27. Which of the following drugs might a type II, or non-insulin-dependent, diabetic take daily to stimulate the production of insulin?

    a. orinase
    b. phenobarbital
    c. dilantin
    d. glucagon

28. Before giving a conscious diabetic an oral glucose solution, you should:

    a. check for a gag reflex
    b. take two sets of vital signs
    c. lay him supine
    d. give him two glasses of water

29. Unconscious hypoglycemic patients may be given intravenous:

    a. glycogen
    b. glucagon
    c. insulin
    d. glucose

30. Anaphylaxis is a serious allergic reaction after patients come into contact with substances to which they have been previously sensitized called:

    a. antigens
    b. antibodies
    c. histamines
    d. antihistamines

31. Shock secondary to anaphylaxis is:

    a. obstructive
    b. cardiogenic
    c. distributive
    d. neurogenic

32. A substance that is released from cells during an anaphylactic reaction that can trigger blood vessels to dilate and capillaries to leak is called:

    a. an antigen
    b. an endorphin
    c. histamine
    d. adrenaline

33. Which of the following is a common agent for producing an anaphylactic reaction?

    a. vegetables
    b. shellfish
    c. milk
    d. fruit

Match the signs and symptoms of anaphylaxis in column B to the physiologic effects in column A.

| Column A | Column B |
|---|---|
| 34. constriction of bronchial smooth muscle | a. hypotension |
| 35. increased permeability of capillaries and fluid leakage | b. swelling of the skin and stridor due to obstruction |
| 36. dilation of the arteries | c. sneezing and nasal congestion |
| 37. increased mucus secretions in the respiratory tree | d. wheezing breath sounds |

38. Some anaphylactic patients may carry a kit that contains antihistamine agents and:

    a. morphine
    b. dilantin
    c. adrenaline
    d. phenobarbital

39. Anaphylactic reactions may present with raised, red patches of skin called:

    a. erythema
    b. purpura
    c. urticaria
    d. papules

40. The major lethal complications of anaphylaxis are circulatory collapse and:

  a. arrhythmias
  b. airway obstruction
  c. heart failure
  d. fluid overload

41. Epinephrine is usually administered subcutaneously at a dose of _____ mg (0.3 ml) of a 1:1000 solution.

  a. 0.3
  b. 1
  c. 2
  d. 5

42. Use of the PSAG in the treatment of shock secondary to anaphylaxis is:

  a. useful to maintain perfusion
  b. contraindicated in all cases
  c. required only if the patient has an airway obstruction
  d. helpful in decreasing the swelling of the extremities

43. HIV infection is transmitted through:

  a. airborne routes
  b. direct contact with infected carrier
  c. urine and fecal exposure
  d. body fluid to body fluid

44. Universal precautions for protection against transmission of HIV and hepatitis B virus when assisting with childbirth include:

  a. gloves and goggles
  b. gloves, goggles and protective clothing
  c. decontaminate site with hypochlorite solution
  d. all of the above

45. All of the following diseases are preventable with vaccines except:

  a. hepatitis B
  b. measles
  c. rubella
  d. tuberculosis

46. Universal precautions are used with all:

    a. AIDS patients
    b. patients
    c. hepatitis patients
    d. infected

47. Diseases capable of being spread from one person to another are called:

    a. syndromes
    b. communicable
    c. endocrine
    d. genetic

48. The precautions one takes to prevent spread of infectious disease are called infection:

    a. control
    b. protection
    c. guarding
    d. barriers

49. The primary national agency that publishes guidelines that help standardize infection control practices across the county is the:

    a. DOH
    b. DOT
    c. CDC
    d. EPA

50. Bacteria, viruses, fungi and parasites are examples of potentially infectious:

    a. invertebrates
    b. microorganisms
    c. arachnids
    d. vertebrates

51. Penicillin is an example of an:

    a. antihistamine
    b. antibiotic
    c. analgesic
    d. anticonvulsant

52. A person, insect, object or other substance that carries or is contaminated by an infectious agent is called a(n):

    a. potent organism
    b. exposer
    c. source
    d. contact

53. A source in which infectious agents can live and multiply, such as a sewer, is called a:

    a. reservoir
    b. container
    c. collecting organism
    d. host

54. The period of time between <u>contact</u> with an infectious agent and occurrence of signs and symptoms is called the _____ period.

    a. incubation
    b. communicable
    c. infectious
    d. development

55. The period during which a person can transmit an infectious disease to others is called the _____ period.

    a. incubation
    b. communicable
    c. infectious
    d. development

56. A person who shows no signs of the disease yet harbors an infectious organism is called a(n):

    a. asymptomatic host
    b. carrier
    c. infector
    d. exposer

57. A term to signify one's coming in contact with, but not necessarily being infected by, a disease-causing agent is:

    a. contact
    b. interface
    c. exposure
    d. casual contact

58.   Infectious disease spread by health care workers or within a health care setting are given the special name:

    a.   health care infections
    b.   treatment-related infections
    c.   nosocomial infections
    d.   provider infections

59.   The direct physical transfer between a susceptible host and an infected or colonized person is referred to as:

    a.   direct transfer
    b.   direct contact
    c.   living contact
    d.   biological contact

60.   Contact of the susceptible host with a contaminated intermediate object, usually inanimate, such as instruments, dressings or other infective material is called:

    a.   passive transfer
    b.   indirect contact
    c.   intermediate contact
    d.   inanimate transfer

61.   Transfer of a microorganism from the spray produced during coughing, sneezing or talking by an infected person is called _____ transmission.

    a.   vapor
    b.   spray
    c.   droplet
    d.   mist

62.   Transmission of a disease through contaminated items, such as transmission of hepatitis (non-A, non-B) by contaminated blood, is a(n) _____ transmission.

    a.   vector
    b.   carrier
    c.   vehicle
    d.   indirect

63.   Transfer of a disease from a mosquito to a person is an example of _____ transmission.

    a.   vector
    b.   carrier
    c.   vehicle
    d.   indirect

64. One's ability to fight off infection following exposure to infectious agents is called:

    a. resistance
    b. organism strength
    c. barrier ability
    d. potentiation

65. The natural antibodies carried by infants that provide protection against many common diseases are called congenital:

    a. resistance
    b. barriers
    c. immunities
    d. protections

66. Injection of microorganisms that are killed or weakened enough to stimulate the immune system, but not enough to cause disease, is called:

    a. passive infection
    b. vaccination
    c. priming
    d. host protection

67. AIDS stands for:

    a. allergic infectious disease syndrome
    b. active infectious disease syndrome
    c. acquired immune deficiency syndrome
    d. active infectious disease syndrome

68. AIDS is transferable via:

    a. indirect contact with objects
    b. body fluid to body fluid contact
    c. skin to skin contact
    d. skin to saliva contact

69. The routine practice of wearing protective clothing (i.e., gloves, goggles) when performing certain procedures (i.e., bleeding control) is called:

    a. general infection prevention
    b. barrier model
    c. immunization
    d. universal precautions

70. The organism that is responsible for AIDS is a:

    a. fungus
    b. bacteria
    c. parasite
    d. virus

71.    AIDS is a disease that compromises the _____ system.

    a.    circulatory
    b.    endocrine
    c.    immune
    d.    central nervous

72.    Modes of transmission for AIDS include all of the following except:

    a.    sexual contact
    b.    needle sharing
    c.    food sharing
    d.    blood transfusion

73.    An infection of the liver caused by one of three different types of viruses is called:

    a.    cirrhosis
    b.    cholecystitis
    c.    gastritis
    d.    hepatitis

74.    The type of hepatitis that is spread by oral and fecal routes is called _____, or infectious hepatitis.

    a.    hepatitis A
    b.    bacterial hepatitis
    c.    hepatitis B
    d.    HBV

75.    The type of hepatitis that is transferred by blood and body fluids is:

    a.    hepatitis A
    b.    bacterial hepatitis
    c.    hepatitis B
    d.    HIV

76.    Which of the following diseases has a vaccination available for prevention?

    a.    AIDS
    b.    hepatitis B
    c.    hepatitis A
    d.    viral meningitis

77. An infection of the covering of the central nervous system that can be caused by viruses, bacteria and other organisms is called:

    a.  encephalitis
    b.  perineuritis
    c.  pleuritis
    d.  meningitis

78. A patient presenting with a recent respiratory infection, fever, headache, stiff neck and altered mental status is most likely suffering from:

    a.  hepatitis
    b.  measles
    c.  meningitis
    d.  pancreatitis

79. Tuberculosis is spread primarily by:

    a.  indirect contact
    b.  vector
    c.  droplets
    d.  blood to blood contact

80. The simplest and most effective measure to block the spread of infections is:

    a.  avoiding physical contact with patients
    b.  using alcohol on infection sites
    c.  handwashing after every patient contact
    d.  wearing a gown with every patient contact

81. When splash from a bleeding artery is possible, the recommended universal precaution is the wearing of:

    a.  mask, goggles and gowns
    b.  mask only
    c.  goggles only
    d.  gown and goggles only

82. The best protection against a needle stick is to:

    a.  wear gloves
    b.  recap all needles
    c.  never recap needles
    d.  use aluminum needles

83. Which of the following solutions is best for cleaning ambulance surfaces after carrying an infectious patient?

    a.  plain soap and water
    b.  hypochlorite solution
    c.  alcohol solution
    d.  pHisoHex solution

84. A regional agency available for phone consultation in the event of a poisoning is called a(n) _____ center.

   a. toxicology
   b. abused substance
   c. poison control
   d. toxic ingestion

Match the substance in column B with the type of poisoning in column A.

| Column A | | Column B | |
|---|---|---|---|
| C 85. | ingestion | a. | carbon monoxide |
| A 86. | inhalation | b. | organophosphates (insecticide) on skin |
| D 87. | injection | c. | methanol |
| B 88. | absorption | d. | scorpion sting |

89. The first priority in the management of an unconscious suspected poison victim is to:

   a. induce vomiting
   b. provide cardiorespiratory support
   c. hasten elimination of the poison
   d. keep the patient awake

90. The three primary questions regarding a poisoning incident are what was taken, how much was taken and:

   a. why it was taken
   b. the age of the patient
   c. whether it was a suicide attempt
   d. when it was taken

91. Prior to inducing vomiting you should:

   a. lay the patient supine
   b. check for a gag reflex
   c. be certain of the exact ingestion dose
   d. administer activated charcoal

92. Inducing vomiting and administering activated charcoal are two methods of:

   a. hastening elimination
   b. neutralizing the poison
   c. preventing absorption
   d. providing an antidote

93.     A cathartic is used to:

        a.    hasten elimination
        b.    neutralize the poison
        c.    reverse the effects of poisons
        d.    induce vomiting

94.     The primary antidote for a carbon monoxide poisoning is:

        a.    carbon dioxide
        b.    naloxone
        c.    oxygen
        d.    cyanide

95.     Patients who have taken an intentional overdose of medication but refuse to go to the hospital:

        a.    have the right to refuse treatment
        b.    may be taken into protective custody
        c.    may be removed only if family approves
        d.    may be removed only after they become unresponsive

96.     The correct dose of syrup of ipecac in an adult is:

        a.    10 ml or two teaspoons
        b.    15 ml or one tablespoon
        c.    30 ml or two tablespoons
        d.    60 ml or four tablespoons

97.     The correct dose of syrup of ipecac for children over 1 year of age is:

        a.    5 ml or one teaspoons
        b.    15 ml or one tablespoon
        c.    30 ml or two tablespoons
        d.    60 ml or four tablespoons

98.     After giving syrup of ipecac to an adult, he or she should also be given:

        a.    activated charcoal immediately
        b.    two glasses of water
        c.    one glass of milk
        d.    an antidote immediately

99.     Which of the following is not a contraindication to inducing vomiting?

        a.    unconsciousness
        b.    corrosive ingestions
        c.    absent gag reflex
        d.    solid material ingestions

100. The universal antidote (burnt toast):

    a. is a potent abortion agent
    b. is better than activated charcoal
    c. should be given just before ipecac
    d. is not used anymore for poisoning

101. The most common pupillary finding in opioid (narcotic) overdoses (i.e., heroin) is:

    a. dilated
    b. midpositional
    c. unequal
    d. pinpoint

102. The major complication of a narcotic overdose is:

    a. arrhythmias
    b. cardiac arrest
    c. respiratory arrest
    d. bleeding

103. Fast heart rates, hypertension, chest pain, anxious behavior, delirium and paranoia best describe an overdose of:

    a. depressants
    b. narcotics
    c. sedative-hypnotics
    d. stimulants

104. Alcohol is a central nervous system:

    a. depressant
    b. stimulant
    c. hypnotic
    d. hallucinogenic

105. A drug that may exhibit little or no symptoms immediately after taken in overdose but which may lead to severe liver failure days later is:

    a. aspirin
    b. Valium
    c. amphetamine
    d. acetaminophen

106. Caustic acid ingestions are best managed in the prehospital phase by administration of:

    a. syrup of ipecac
    b. two glasses of milk or water
    c. neutralizing agents
    d. soda solution

107. The <u>first</u> and most important step in the management of an inhalation poisoning is:

    (a.) removal from the toxic environment
    b. administration of oxygen
    c. positive pressure ventilation
    d. cardiopulmonary resuscitation

108. Gases that react with water in the lungs and primarily cause inflammatory damage to the airway and bronchoconstriction are called:

    a. asphyxiants
    (b.) irritants
    c. organophosphates
    d. chemical asphyxiants

109. Eyes that have be exposed to corrosive chemicals should be irrigated for a minimum of:

    a. 2-3 minutes
    b. 5-10 minutes
    c. 10-15 minutes
    (d.) 15-20 minutes

110. All of the following are commonly injected drugs <u>except</u>:

    a. amphetamine
    (b.) acetaminophen
    c. cocaine
    d. heroin

Match the type of snake in column B with the distinguishing features in column A.

| Column A | Column B |
| --- | --- |
| B 111. elliptical eyes | a. nonpoisonous |
| A 112. round eyes | b. pit vipers |
| B 113. pit between eyes and nostrils | |
| B 114. fangs | |
| B 115. triangular head | |

116. In the treatment of poisonous snakebites, attempts to suck out the venom:

   a.   are required in every case
   b.   remove 90% of the venom
   c.   are highly controversial
   d.   should be done after swelling occurs

117. Which of the following is a useful technique to minimize distribution of the poison of a snakebite?

   a.   immobilizing the affected part
   b.   applying an arterial tourniquet
   c.   6 ounces of alcohol
   d.   placing the part on ice

## Case Histories

| Case History #1 |
| --- |
| You respond to an office an find a 35 year old man who is extremely combative and who appears psychotic.  His coworkers advise you that he is normally a mild-mannered guy and suddenly he became aggressive for no reason. While you are evaluating the situation, he becomes quiet and lethargic and you note that he is pale, cool and sweaty.  His vital signs are pulse 110 and regular, blood pressure 140/90, and respirations 24 and regular.  A medic alert tag identifies him as a diabetic. |

118. Based on the description, you suspect:

   a.   diabetic ketoacidosis
   b.   hypoglycemia
   c.   hyperglycemia
   d.   hyperosmolar coma

119. Your immediate action should be to:

   a.   give him something sweet to drink
   b.   provide deep pain stimulus to keep him awake
   c.   transport only
   d.   give him insulin tablets

120. Before taking the above action, you should check for:

   a.   identification
   b.   a gag reflex
   c.   track marks
   d.   urticaria

121. The above condition was most likely caused by:

    a.     forgetting to take insulin
    b.     eating too much sugar
    c.     not eating at the proper time
    d.     taking too little insulin

---

**Case History #2**

You respond to a call and find a 58 year old man unresponsive to painful stimuli in his bed at home. He was last seen by his son 2 days ago. Physical exam reveals pale dry skin, dilated pupils and deep and rapid breathing. You note a fruity smell on his breath. His vital signs are pulse 120 and thready, respirations 28 and deep, and blood pressure 90/60. While you are assessing him, the patient begins to vomit.

---

122. Based on the description you suspect:

    a.     diabetic ketoacidosis
    b.     hypoglycemia
    c.     hyperglycemia
    d.     hyperosmolar coma

123. Your immediate action should include all of the following, <u>except:</u>

    a.     turning him on to his left side and suction
    b.     providing high concentration oxygen
    c.     giving him a sugar solution by mouth
    d.     rapid transport

124. The breathing pattern is the body's attempt to:

    a.     gain more oxygen
    b.     blow off acid
    c.     blow off sugar
    d.     decrease temperature

125. The hypotension is most likely the result of:

    a.     vasodilation
    b.     dehydration
    c.     acidosis
    d.     cardiac failure

---

## Case History #3

You respond to a call for "difficulty breathing." Upon arrival you find a 16 year old boy who is unresponsive and who appears cyanotic on the lips and nail beds. Physical exam reveals pale sweaty skin, with cyanosis around the lips and nailbeds, and red, raised areas of skin around the body. You note swelling of the tongue and facial and neck tissues, and the patient is experiencing stridor. Breath sounds reveal wheezing throughout the lungs fields. Vital signs are pulse 130 and thready, respirations 32 with accessary muscle use and retractions, and blood pressure 80/60.

---

126.  Based on the description, you suspect:

  a.  foreign body airway obstruction
  b.  asthma
  c.  bronchitis
  d.  anaphylaxis

127.  Your actions should include all of the following except:

  a.  applying abdominal thrusts
  b.  positive pressure ventilation
  c.  applying the PASG
  d.  rapid transport

128.  The stridor is related to:

  a.  the foreign body
  b.  bronchiole constriction
  c.  swelling of the upper airway
  d.  thickening of the tracheal mucosa

129.  The hypotension is most likely the result of:

  a.  vasodilation
  b.  hypoxia
  c.  obstruction
  d.  cardiac failure

130.  The definitive treatment for this condition includes:

  a.  dilantin
  b.  phenobarbital
  c.  epinephrine
  d.  glucagon

131. If this patient were to develop a complete obstruction on the way to the hospital, your best action would be:

    a. abdominal thrusts
    b. finger sweeps
    c. suctioning
    (d.) forced positive pressure

---

### Case History #4

You respond to a poisoning and find a 5 year old girl who is suspected of a having ingested 100 acetaminophen (Tylenol) tablets 10 minutes earlier. The mother shows you an empty bottle, but the child appears perfectly normal and has normal vital signs. The child is alert and oriented.

---

132. Normal vital signs in this type of overdose are:

    a. possible but not likely
    (b.) likely in the first 24 hours
    c. possible only in the first few minutes
    d. highly unlikely after 5 minutes

133. You contact poison control for advise. What do you think they will most likely advise as a first step under these circumstances?

    (a.) give 15 ml (1 tablespoon) of ipecac
    b. give several glasses of water
    c. give activated charcoal
    d. rapid transport only

134. Had she ingested Drano, what would the likely treatment be?

    a. give 15 ml (1 tablespoon) of ipecac
    (b.) give 1 or 2 glasses of water or milk
    c. give activated charcoal
    d. rapid transport only

---

### Case History #5

You respond to a call and find 50 year old man locked in his garage with his car motor running. He is unresponsive and has a bright cherry red skin color.

---

135. Your immediate action should be to:

    a.  open the garage door, turn off the car engine and give high concentration oxygen
    b.  remove the patient from the garage and give high concentration oxygen
    c.  immediately transport the patient to the hospital to be intubated
    d.  give humidified oxygen via nasal cannula and transport

136. The cherry red color is from:

    a.  unsaturated hemoglobin
    b.  hemoglobin saturated with carbon dioxide
    c.  hemoglobin saturated with carbon monoxide
    d.  hemoglobin saturated with cyanide

137. The antidote for this poisoning is:

    a.  amyl nitrate
    b.  nitrous oxide
    c.  oxygen
    d.  naloxone

138. Which of the following definitive treatments would be most helpful for this patient?

    a.  hyperbaric oxygen
    b.  intubation and ventilation
    c.  heart-lung machine
    d.  dialysis

---

### Case History #6

While on stand-by at an EMS picnic, you are called for a snakebite case. A 24 year old male was bitten in the ankle by a snake, and his associate killed the snake just prior to your arrival.

---

139. You examine the snake and note elliptical eyes, a pit between the eyes and nose, and a triangular head. You conclude that the snake is:

    a.  poisonous
    b.  not poisonous
    c.  poisonous only if it is brightly colored
    d.  poisonous only if it has a rattle tail

140. Your response time to a hospital will be approximately 1 hour. Which of the following actions is appropriate under these conditions?

    a.    apply ice to the ankle
    b.    apply an arterial tourniquet
    c.    apply an elastic bandage and immobilize the limb
    d.    cut an X and suck out the venom

---

### Case History #7

You respond to an overdose and find a 22 year old male with track marks on his arm and who is unresponsive to painful stimuli. Physical exam reveals pinpointed pupils, and snoring is heard with each breath. His vital signs are respirations 10 and shallow, pulse 62 and thready, and blood pressure 90/60.

---

141. Your immediate action is to:

    a.    open the airway and begin positive pressure ventilation
    b.    suction and administer oxygen via nasal cannula
    c.    apply the PASG
    d.    induce vomiting

142. What universal precautions are appropriate for this patient?

    a.    gloves only
    b.    gown and gloves only
    c.    goggles, gloves and gown
    d.    none are needed

143. Based on the signs and symptoms you suspect:

    a.    amphetamine overdose
    b.    barbiturate overdose
    c.    opiate overdose
    d.    sedative-hynotic overdose

---

### Case History #8

You find a 22 year old girl at home in bed who is responsive to painful but not verbal stimuli. She has a fever, and her sister advises you that she had an upper respiratory infection and a severe headache prior to becoming unresponsive. Physical exam reveals a stiff neck and very hot skin.

---

144. Based on the signs and symptoms you suspect:

    a.    pneumonia
    b.    meningitis
    c.    subarachnoid hemorrhage
    d.    encephalitis

145. What contact with this patient is most hazardous?

    a.    patient's respiratory secretions to your mouth
    b.    patient's skin to your skin
    c.    patient's blood to your skin
    d.    patient's urine to your skin

Chapter 12

Skill Performance Sheet

# Inducing Vomiting with Syrup of Ipecac

Student Name_____          Date_____

| Performance Standard | Performed | Failed |
|---|---|---|
| Check that the patient is responsive | | |
| Check for a gag reflex | | |
| Administer ipecac:<br>(adult, 30ml; child over 1, 15ml) | | |
| Administer 1-2 glasses of water | | |
| Place patient in sitting position | | |
| Have suction at the ready | | |
| Transport and observe | | |

Comments_____

_____

_____

_____

Instructor _____          Circle One:  Pass  Fail

## Chapter 13

# OBSTETRICAL AND GYNECOLOGIC EMERGENCIES

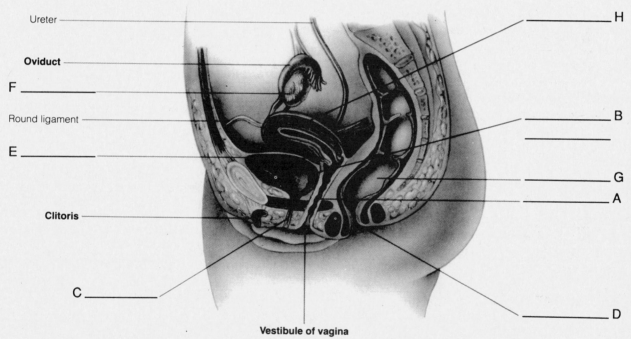

(Gaudin AJ, Jones KC: Human Anatomy and Physiology. Harcourt Brace Jovanovich, Publishers 1989 pg 709.)

Match the structures above to the terms below.

C 1. urethra

H 2. uterus

F 3. cervix

F 4. ovary

A 5. vagina

B 6. urinary bladder

G 7. rectum

D 8. anus

*Chapter 13*

Match the answer in column A with the best symptoms or definition from column B.

| Column A | | Column B | |
|---|---|---|---|
| D 9. | missed abortion | a. | missed period and sudden onset of abdominal pain often referred to shoulder with vaginal bleeding and signs of shock |
| F 10. | pelvic inflammatory disease (PID) | b. | marked by sharp, tearing pain and an abrupt cessation of labor pains |
| E 11. | abruptio placenta | | |
| C 12. | placenta previa | c. | painless, bright red vaginal bleeding |
| G 13. | disseminated intravascular coagulation (DIC) | d. | dead fetus retained in uterus |
| B 14. | ruptured uterus | e. | rigid uterus, bleeding may be dark, no break between contractions |
| A 15. | ruptured ectopic pregnancy | | |
| | | f. | fever, abdominal pain and vaginal discharge |
| | | g. | disruption of the normal clotting mechanism with uncontrollable hemorrhage as a result |

16. What is the largest diameter of the pelvic outlet?

    a. transverse
    b. anteroposterior
    c. oblique
    d. lateral

17. The release of a mature egg from the female ovary is called:

    a. menstruation
    b. conception
    c. fertilization
    d. ovulation

18.    A major function of the fallopian tubes is the:

       a.    carries eggs from ovary to the uterus
       b.    site of implantation of a normal pregnancy
       c.    connecting point between the cervix and the vagina
       d.    site of egg production

19.    The part of the body where eggs are stored and become mature and where
       female hormones are produced is the:

       a.    fallopian tube
       b.    uterus
       c.    ovary
       d.    cervix

20.    The section of the uterus that must be effaced and dilated during labor is the:

       a.    body
       b.    cervix
       c.    fundus
       d.    myometrium

21.    The lining of the uterus into which the embryo implants and that is shed
       during menstruation is the:

       a.    myometrium
       b.    endometrium
       c.    perimetrium
       d.    cervometrium

22.    The uppermost part of the uterus is the:

       a.    cervix
       b.    fundus
       c.    endometrium
       d.    crown

23.    The organ through which nutrients and waste products are exchanged
       between the baby and the mother is the:

       a.    uterus
       b.    placenta
       c.    liver
       d.    cervix

24.    The umbilical cord contains:

       a.    one vein and one artery
       b.    one vein and two arteries
       c.    two veins and one artery
       d.    two veins and two arteries

25. The first stage of labor:

    a. begins with full dilation of the cervix and ends when the baby is born
    b. lasts from the onset of contractions until the cervix is completely dilated
    c. ends at the onset of transition
    d. should never last more than 1 hour

26. In the transition period of labor, you can expect:

    a. contractions 2-3 minutes apart lasting 60-90 seconds
    b. sweating and nausea
    c. delivery of the placenta
    d. a and b only
    e. all of the above

27. True labor is differentiated from false labor by:

    a. intensity of contractions
    b. regularity of contractions
    c. dilation of the cervix
    d. amount of bloody show

28. All of the following are parts of the mechanism of childbirth <u>except</u>:

    a. flexion
    b. composition
    c. internal rotation
    d. expulsion

29. During the second stage of labor:

    a. the mother often has an urge to move her bowels
    b. postpartum hemorrhage may occur
    c. you can expect to deliver the placenta
    d. labor contractions stop

30. During a normal vertex delivery, as soon as the baby's head is born, you should:

    a. immediately tell the mother to push before the cervix closes
    b. ask the mother to pant while you check to see if there is a cord wrapped around the baby's neck
    c. examine the baby's mouth to see if he or she has a cleft lip
    d. dry the baby's head

31.    Your <u>first</u> action after the baby is out is to:

    a.     clamp the cord
    b.     suction the baby's mouth and nose with a bulb syringe
    c.     dry the baby thoroughly
    d.     deliver the placenta

32.    If a baby's head is born and you find that the umbilical cord is wrapped tightly around the baby's neck, you should:

    a.     give the mother oxygen and transport rapidly
    b.     stretch the cord over the baby's head to unwind it
    c.     clamp the cord close together in two places and cut between the clamps
    d.     try to push the head back inside a little bit to ease tension around the baby's neck

33.    McRobert's maneuver, sharply flexing the mother's knees back toward either side of her abdomen, straightens the spine and may be useful:

    a.     when the placenta will not deliver
    b.     in the pregnant trauma victim
    c.     when the head is born but the shoulders seem to be stuck
    d.     in a postpartum hemorrhage

34.    In a vertex delivery with meconium-stained fluid, the mouth should be suctioned:

    a.     only after the nose is suctioned
    b.     as soon as the head is born, before delivering the rest of the baby
    c.     only after you check the heart rate
    d.     the mouth should not be suctioned because you will contaminate the mouth with bacteria

35.    When you find that the baby's leg is projecting out of the vagina in a laboring patient, you should:

    a.     grasp the leg firmly and pull until you can reach the other leg
    b.     transport rapidly while giving oxygen to the mother
    c.     try to push the leg back inside the vagina
    d.     press on the mother's fundus and ask her to push

36.    After a baby is born and the cord is cut, you notice a sudden gush of about 50 ml of blood from the mother's vagina and lengthening of the umbilical cord. This would indicate:

    a.     laceration of the vagina
    b.     the onset of a postpartum hemorrhage
    c.     the placenta is about to deliver
    d.     uterine rupture

37. Allowing the mother to nurse a healthy, full-term newborn after birth:

   a. should never be done in the ambulance
   b. can help to contract the uterus
   c. can relieve cyanosis in a newborn
   d. supplies the baby with the calories it needs

38. If the placenta does not spontaneously deliver within 15-20 minutes after the baby is born, you should:

   a. ask the mother to push while you pull on the cord
   b. proceed to the hospital
   c. ask the mother to stand; gravity may deliver the placenta
   d. perform McRobert's maneuver

39. All of the following are normal in the newborn except:

   a. a heart rate of 156
   b. a white, creamy film on the baby's skin
   c. tiny white spots covering the nose and chin
   d. limpness or apparent weakness in one or both arms

40. When resuscitating a newborn, the heart rate is counted for:

   a. a full minute
   b. 6 seconds
   c. only after the Apgar score is done
   d. 30 seconds

41. All the following are symptoms of respiratory distress in the newborn except:

   a. grunting
   b. nasal flaring
   c. cyanosis of the hands and feet
   d. sternal retractions

42. All of the following are improper actions when resuscitating a newborn except:

   a. hyperextending the neck before ventilating
   b. quickly drying the baby immediately after birth
   c. giving chest compressions with the heel of one hand
   d. ventilating the baby at a rate of 80 breaths/min

43. Positive pressure ventilation for a newborn should be done at a rate of:

   a. 20-30 breaths/min
   b. 40-60 breaths/min
   c. 80-100 breaths/min
   d. 120-140 breaths/min

44. The concentration of oxygen for positive pressure ventilation of a newborn should be:

    a. 90-100%
    b. 40-50%
    c. never give oxygen to a newborn

45. Chest compressions in the newborn should be:

    a. 1/2-3/4 inch at 100 beats/min
    b. 1/2-3/4 inch at 120 beats/min
    c. 1-2 inch at 150 beats/min
    d. 1-2 inch at 120 beats/min

46. A newborn is breathing at birth, so you check the heart rate. It is 85. Your next action would be to:

    a. evaluate the baby's color
    b. begin positive pressure ventilation with 100% oxygen
    c. begin cardiac compressions
    d. give 100% free-flow oxygen

47. When resuscitating a newborn, cardiac compressions should be discontinued once the baby's heart rate has reached:

    a. 50
    b. 80
    c. 90-100
    d. compressions should not be performed at all if the baby has a heart rate

48. An infant born with a cleft palate:

    a. will probably also be brain damaged
    b. should not be allowed to nurse
    c. should not be shown to the mother
    d. all of the above

49. Allowing the newborn to become chilled can:

    a. help to establish respirations if the baby does not cry
    b. cause hypoglycemia and acidosis
    c. stimulate a more rapid heart rate as the baby tries to stay warm
    d. help to keep the baby awake so that it can nurse

50.   A common complication of abdominal trauma in the pregnant patient is:

    a.   placenta previa
    b.   ruptured bowel
    c.   abruptio placenta
    d.   all of the above

51.   In general, the position for transport of a pregnant patient in her third trimester is:

    a.   supine
    b.   prone
    c.   on her left side
    d.   on her right side

52.   The reason for transporting a pregnant woman on her left side is:

    a.   you always want to have the mother facing you in the ambulance
    b.   most babies are facing the mother's right side late in pregnancy, and pressure on the back of the babies head can dangerously lower the heart rate
    c.   to prevent damage to the liver
    d.   the vena cava is right of the midline and you do not want to compress it between the spinal column and the weight of the baby

53.   During normal pregnancy, the blood pressure:

    a.   should not change
    b.   becomes slightly higher than it was before pregnancy
    c.   becomes much higher than it was before pregnancy
    d.   becomes lower than it was before pregnancy

54.   A baby born to a diabetic mother:

    a.   is prone to hypoglycemia after delivery
    b.   is prone to hyperglycemia after delivery
    c.   is not usually affected by the mother's disease
    d.   will probably be born with diabetes

55.   A baby born to a diabetic mother is likely to be:

    a.   larger than normal
    b.   smaller than normal
    c.   average size

56.   Maternal hypertension is defined as:

    a.   systolic greater than 180 or diastolic greater than 100
    b.   systolic greater than 160 or diastolic greater than 100
    c.   systolic greater than 150 or diastolic greater than 90
    d.   systolic greater than 140 or diastolic greater than 90

57.     Preeclampsia becomes eclampsia when:

    a.      hypertension and edema are both present
    b.      the blood pressure exceeds 180/100
    c.      a seizure occurs
    d.      all of the above

58.     All of the following are predisposing factors to ectopic pregnancy except:

    a.      history of PID
    b.      previous ectopic
    c.      tubal ligation
    d.      high blood pressure

59.     If you examine a laboring patient and find the umbilical cord bulging out of the vagina, you should:

    a.      clamp and cut the cord so that the baby can be delivered
    b.      try to elevate the presenting part with a gloved hand so it does not compress the cord
    c.      gently place the cord back inside the vagina
    d.      place a moist pressure dressing over the vagina

60.     Prolapsed cord is often associated with:

    a.      placenta previa
    b.      abruptio placenta
    c.      abnormal presentation, such as breech or shoulder
    d.      preeclampsia

## Case Histories

### Case History #1

You arrive at a call to find a patient who states she is approximately 32 week's pregnant, but she has not seen a doctor because she has no money. She awoke in the middle of the night and was very upset to find that she had passed a good deal of bright red blood from her vagina. She has no abdominal or pelvic tenderness, but complains of mild low back pain. Her skin is pale, warm and dry to the touch. Her vital signs are blood pressure 100/56, pulse 108 and respirations 22.

61.     The most likely cause of this patient's vaginal bleeding is:

    a.      abruption of the placenta
    b.      ruptured uterus
    c.      placenta previa
    d.      the patient is about to deliver shortly

62. Your first action at this time would be to:

    a. do a gentle vaginal exam to see if the patient is about to deliver
    b. place the patient on her left side and give high concentration oxygen
    c. insert a pressure dressing into the vagina to control the bleeding
    d. massage the patient's uterus to control the bleeding

63. The use of PASG for this patient is:

    a. not indicated given her presentation
    b. a good idea if she is still actively loosing a large amount of blood, but the abdominal compartment should not be inflated
    c. a good idea if she is actively loosing a large amount of blood; all compartments should be inflated

---

### Case History #2

You arrive at a call to find a woman who is 30 week's pregnant with her second child. She complains of labor pains but cannot say how far apart they are because the pain is almost constant. Her uterus feels hard and she is restless and crying with the pains. History reveals that she was in a motor vehicle accident yesterday, was seen in the emergency room and treated for sprained wrists, which she injured bracing herself against the dashboard. She was a front seat passenger wearing a lap belt restraint. There is no vaginal bleeding or discharge. Her vital signs are blood pressure 130/80, pulse 114 and respirations 24.

---

64. This patient's constant labor pain alerts you to the possibility that she probably has:

    a. preeclampsia
    b. premature labor
    c. abruptio placenta
    d. ruptured membranes

65. Your best action at this time would be to:

    a. take out an obstetric kit and prepare for a premature delivery
    b. place her on her left side, give oxygen and transport immediately
    c. do a vaginal exam to see if the cervix is dilated
    d. use McRobert's maneuver

---

### Case History #3

A patient complains of severe shoulder pain that came on suddenly. Physical exam reveals abdominal tenderness, and she is starting to experience some vaginal bleeding. Her skin is pale, cool and clammy. She missed her last period.

---

66.     This patient's symptoms are most likely caused by:

   a.     placenta previa
   b.     threatened abortion
   c.     ruptured ectopic pregnancy
   d.     breech presentation

67.     The patient's history reveals all of the following information. Which fact is the most common predisposing factor related to her current condition?

   a.     she was hospitalized for pelvic inflammatory disease last year
   b.     she takes medication for high blood pressure
   c.     she had a baby 5 years ago, and the pregnancy was complicated by placenta previa
   d.     she is an insulin-dependent diabetic

---

### Case History #4

You arrive at a call to find a patient in labor. She is very uncomfortable, with contractions occurring every 3 minutes and lasting 60 seconds. She is noisy and restless with contractions and loudly demands to go to the bathroom. Physical exam reveals a slight bulging of the perineum and rectum, but no presenting part is visible. There is a gush of fluid during a contraction, and you note that the fluid is meconium stained.

---

68.     The meconium in the fluid alerts you to all of the following except:

   a.     the baby may be breech
   b.     there is a 20% chance that the baby may have respiratory distress
   c.     the fetus has had a bowel movement
   d.     the mother probably has an infection

69.     Your best action at this time would be to:

   a.     explain that the urge to go to the bathroom is probably the baby coming, then have the woman lie on her bed and prepare for a delivery
   b.     allow her to go to the bathroom so that she will be more cooperative
   c.     explain that the urge to go to the bathroom is probably the baby coming, then get her to lie on the stretcher in the ambulance and prepare for a delivery enroute to the hospital
   d.     put the mother in knee-chest position

---

### Case History #5

You arrive at a call and find a 34 year old woman who has just delivered her third child, a full-term female. A survey of the newborn reveals a healthy infant with well-established respirations, and no signs of distress. The placenta delivers spontaneously, and you are about to transfer when the vaginal bleeding becomes very heavy. Her blood pressure is 90/50, pulse is 118, and respirations are 22. Her skin is cool, somewhat clammy and pale.

---

70.   The most common cause of <u>early</u> postpartum hemorrhage is:

      a.     perineal lacerations
      b.     uterine atony
      c.     ruptured uterus
      d.     prolapsed uterus

71.   Your <u>first</u> action would be to:

      a.     apply direct pressure to the perineum
      b.     palpate and massage the uterus
      c.     elevate the patient's hips
      d.     apply an ice pack to the perineum

72.   Postpartum hemorrhage is defined as a blood loss equal to or greater than

      a.     100 ml
      b.     500 ml
      c.     800 ml
      d.     1000 ml

---

### Case History #6

You arrive at a call to find a 19 year old female who has been beaten and raped by a stranger. Her clothes are torn and bloodstained, and she is crying.

---

73.   The best way to proceed in this situation is:

      a.     gently help the woman to change her clothes, wash up and transport
      b.     gently assess for further injuries, treat as necessary and transport
      c.     examine her perineum to assess for injuries
      d.     encourage her to douche before you go to the hospital to prevent infection

74.   The best attitude to take with this patient is to:

      a.     minimize the event so that it does not seem so bad
      b.     be gentle, understanding and compassionate
      c.     talk to her as little as possible
      d.     be authoritative, since she needs to feel someone is in control

---

**Case History #7**

You have a patient whose chief complaints are epigastric pain, headache and dizziness. She is about 30 week's pregnant and has marked puffiness in her hands, legs and face. As you lift the stretcher, she starts to complain of blurred vision. Her vital signs are blood pressure 170/100, pulse 122 and respirations 24.

---

75.  This patient is probably suffering from:

   a.  diabetes
   b.  heart attack
   c.  preeclampsia
   d.  gastric ulcer

76.  Your best action at this time would be to:

   a.  put on lights and sirens and rush to the hospital
   b.  place her on her left side, give oxygen, have suction equipment ready and proceed quietly to the hospital
   c.  ask her to push so you can deliver the baby
   d.  give her milk to drink to relieve the gastric acidity

77.  The dizziness, blurred vision and headache are probably caused by:

   a.  cerebral and retinal edema
   b.  gastric ulcer
   c.  hypoglycemia
   d.  shock

78.  There is a good possibility that this patient may soon suffer from a:

   a.  cardiac arrest
   b.  full gastric bleed
   c.  seizure
   d.  hypoglycemic reaction

---

**Case History #8**

You arrive at an obstetrical call to find that a breech delivery is in progress. The baby has been born up to the neck.

---

79.  The head of a breech baby is most likely to become stuck in which of the following?

   a.  a 7 pound, 42 week gestation baby
   b.  a 6 pound, 40 week gestation baby
   c.  a 7 pound, 38 week gestation baby
   d.  a 5 pound, 30 week gestation baby

80. Which of the following is almost always present in a breech delivery?

    a.    a premature baby
    b.    meconium fluid
    c.    an umbilical cord around the neck
    d.    heavy vaginal bleeding

81. The mother is pushing uncontrollably, but the head will not deliver. To assist, you might:

    a.    twist the baby's body around until the head pops out
    b.    place two fingers up into the baby's mouth and flex the baby's chin onto his chest
    c.    clamp and cut the umbilical cord
    d.    place the mother on her left side and ask her to stop pushing

82. After the baby is born, you hand him to your partner. He quickly dries the baby off and positions him on a clean towel. The next action should be to:

    a.    thoroughly suction the baby's mouth and then the nose
    b.    stimulate the baby to cry by firmly slapping the soles of his feet
    c.    do an Apgar score
    d.    check the baby's heart rate

83. The baby requires the use of positive pressure ventilation. The percentage of oxygen given during positive pressure ventilation of this baby is:

    a.    100%
    b.    80%
    c.    50%
    d.    21%

84. After 30 seconds of positive pressure ventilation, your partner checks the baby's heart rate. It is 70. He should now:

    a.    discontinue positive pressure ventilation
    b.    continue positive pressure ventilation and begin chest compressions
    c.    stimulate the baby if it is breathing
    d.    suction the baby

85. The baby has been successfully resuscitated. You notice that his right arm hangs limply at his side and there is no grasp reflex in the hand. This is probably due to:

    a.    brain damage
    b.    damage to the brachial nerves
    c.    hypoglycemia
    d.    dislocation of the shoulder

86.     Your best action at this time would be to:

a.      reduce the dislocation by pulling the arm out and then up

b.      immobilize the arm by wrapping the baby firmly in a blanket and handling it as little as possible

c.      continue to stimulate the baby's hand until you can elicit a grasp reflex

d.      wrap the baby loosely with the arm outside the blanket and ask the mother to nurse the baby

Skill Performance Sheet

## Normal Childbirth

Student Name_____          Date_____

| Performance Standard | Performed | Failed |
|---|---|---|
| EMT #1 washes hands, if possible | | |
| Apply gloves using sterile technique and prepare sterile field | | |
| Apply gentle pressure on baby's head with flat hand | | |
| Once head is delivered, check for cord around baby's neck | | |
| If cord cannot be slipped over the head, clamp and cut cord if around neck | | |
| Suction mouth if there is meconium-stained fluid | | |
| Ask mother to push and gently deliver shoulders with downward traction for upper shoulder and upward traction for lower shoulder | | |
| Suction baby with bulb syringe | | |
| Place baby on dry towels | | |
| Deliver placenta | | |
| Massage uterus as necessary | | |
| Place placenta in bag | | |
| Deliver mother and baby to hospital while keeping warm | | |

Comments_____

_____

Instructor _____          Circle One:   Pass   Fail

Skill Performance Sheet

**Resuscitation of the Newborn**

Student Name_____          Date_____

| Performance Standard | Performed | Failed |
|---|---|---|
| Dry infant and place on clean towel in a warm place | | |
| Place head in "sniffing position" | | |
| Suction mouth and nose with bulb syringe | | |
| Evaluate breathing | | |
| If not breathing, stimulate infant by rubbing back and slapping feet | | |
| If not breathing, provide positive pressure ventilation (40/min) | | |
| Evaluate heart rate after 30 seconds of ventilation | | |
| If heart rate is less than 80, begin chest compressions at a rate of 120 compressions per minute | | |
| If heart rate is between 80-100, continue positive pressure ventilation, but do not perform compressions | | |
| After 30 seconds of chest compression, check heart rate | | |
| If below 80, continue CPR | | |

Comments_____

_____

_____

_____

Instructor _____          Circle One:   Pass   Fail

## Chapter 14

### PEDIATRIC EMERGENCIES

1.    The most common cause of death in children outside of the newborn period
      is:

      a.    SIDS
      b.    accidents and respiratory conditions
      c.    congenital heart disease
      d.    cancer

2.    Most cardiopulmonary arrests in children result from failure of the
      _____ system.

      a.    urinary
      b.    cardiovascular
      c.    respiratory
      d.    endocrine

3.    Magical thinking is primarily associated with which of the following periods
      of development?

      a.    infants--less than 1 year
      b.    toddlers--15 months to 3 years
      c.    small children--4-7 years
      d.    adolescents

4.    When examining adolescents it is most important to:

      a.    respect their privacy and shyness
      b.    relax them with casual conversation
      c.    be assertive to avoid resistance to questions
      d.    be upbeat and familiar with them

5.    When examining small children it is a good idea to:

      a.    ask the parents to leave the room
      b.    hold them on your lap
      c.    leave them on their parents' laps
      d.    do it quickly to avoid problems

6.    In small children the secondary survey should proceed:

      a.    in the same manner as in an adult
      b.    in a toe to head structure
      c.    briskly to avoid prolonged exposure
      d.    very slowly to avoid agitation

7.  The narrowest part of the upper airway in infants is the:

    a.  epiglottis
    b.  trachea
    c.  thyroid cartilage
    d.  cricoid cartilage

8.  To open the airway of the infant, place the head in the
    _____ position.

    a.  hyperflexed
    b.  extended
    c.  flexed
    d.  sniffing or neutral

9.  Hyperextension of an infant's airway may result in:

    a.  kinking and obstruction
    b.  rupture of the larynx
    c.  dislocation of the cervical spine
    d.  increased intracranial pressure

10. Infants (up to 1 year) have an average respiratory rate of approximately
    _____ breaths per minute.

    a.  12-20
    b.  20-25
    c.  24-30
    d.  30-40

11. Infants breath dominantly through the:

    a.  nose
    b.  mouth
    c.  pursed lips
    d.  cheeks

12. During ventilation you must be careful to closely observe _____ to
    determine the effectiveness of ventilation.

    a.  pupil response
    b.  skin color
    c.  capillary refill
    d.  chest rise

13. When ventilating an infant, care should be taken not to over-ventilate since infants are more subject to _____ than adults.

    a. pneumothorax
    b. gastric distention
    c. hemothorax
    d. pulmonary contusions

14. Nasal flaring and retractions are signs of _____ in an infant.

    a. increased work of breathing
    b. difficulty with exhalation
    c. chest wall injury
    d. hyperventilation

15. High concentration oxygen therapy for children over 1 year of age:

    a. is contraindicated
    b. may cause blindness
    c. is appropriate if needed
    d. is never needed

16. As a general rule, the width of a blood pressure cuff applied to an infant or child should cover approximately _____ of the length of the upper arm

    a. 1/4
    b. 1/3
    c. 2/3
    d. 1/2

17. The American College of Surgeons considers a systolic blood pressure of less than _____ mm Hg with tachycardia and cool skin an indicator of shock in children.

    a. 50
    b. 70
    c. 80
    d. 90

18. Infants and children have a _____ baseline metabolic rate than adults.

    a. higher
    b. lower

19. Early signs of dehydration in children include all of the following except:

    a. tachycardia
    b. decreased urination
    c. dry mucosal membranes
    d. hypotension

20. Because of their healthier compensatory mechanisms, children maintain their blood pressure until nearly _____ of blood volume is lost.

    a.    20%
    b.    30%
    c.    40%
    d.    50%

21. A crowing, high pitched sound made on inspiration that is suggestive of upper airway obstruction is called:

    a.    grunting
    b.    snoring
    c.    wheezing
    d.    stridor

22. A rhythmic sound heard at the end of exhalation that may be mistaken for whining is called:

    a.    grunting
    b.    snoring
    c.    wheezing
    d.    stridor

23. The inward depression of muscular areas and their attached ribs, which are drawn inward and reflect an increased work at breathing, is called:

    a.    thoracic paradoxis
    b.    myotonia
    c.    retractions
    d.    myopia

24. High pitched "musical" sounds caused by narrowing of the lower airways obstructing airflow is called:

    a.    rales
    b.    stridor
    c.    wheezing
    d.    grunting

25. All of the following are common causes of upper airway obstruction in infants and small children except:

    a.    bronchitis
    b.    croup
    c.    foreign bodies
    d.    epiglottitis

26. A viral infection affecting the larynx, trachea and bronchi that can cause airway narrowing, especially at the level of the cricoid ring, is called:

    a. bronchiolitis
    b. pharyngitis
    c. croup
    d. epiglottitis

27. All of the following are signs of the condition described above <u>except</u>:

    a. a hoarse voice
    b. wheezing
    c. a barking cough
    d. a low-grade fever

28. Croup is most common from ages _____, with the majority of cases occurring at less than 3 years old.

    a. 6 months to 6 years
    b. newborn to 4 years
    c. 1 year to 8 years
    d. newborn to 11 years

29. The effective management of croup includes all of the following <u>except</u>:

    a. positioning the child supine
    b. oxygenation
    c. humidification
    d. hydration in the hospital

30. Epiglottitis is an acute bacterial infection of the epiglottis that has a rapid onset of approximately _____ hours.

    a. 2-4
    b. 1-2
    c. 10-12
    d. 24-72

31. Which of the following is not a common sign of acute epiglottitis?

    a. high fever
    b. sore throat
    c. difficulty in swallowing
    d. absent breath sounds on one side

32.   The child with epiglottitis will frequently be sitting upright and leaning forward resting the chin on the arms.  This is called the _____ position.

      a.   Fowler
      b.   recumbent
      c.   semi-Fowler
      d.   tripod

33.   A major contraindication in the management of acute epiglottitis is:

      a.   administering high-concentration oxygen
      b.   examining the pharynx with a tongue blade
      c.   humidifying oxygen during administration
      d.   none of the above

34.   When faced with a child who has a complete airway obstruction due to acute epiglottitis or croup, you should:

      a.   administer back blows and chest thrusts
      b.   attempt forced ventilation with the BVM
      c.   initiate rapid transport
      d.   both b and c

35.   A child with a foreign body airway obstruction who is alert and demonstrating effective air exchange should be managed by:

      a.   a deep finger sweep to the upper airway
      b.   back blows and chest thrusts
      c.   transport only
      d.   positive pressure ventilation

36.   The correct management of a conscious, complete foreign body airway obstruction in an infant is:

      a.   back blows
      b.   chest thrusts
      c.   finger sweep
      d.   both a and b

37.   The correct position for an infant while administering back blows is:

      a.   supporting the head in your hand
      b.   resting on your arm and thigh
      c.   the head in the dependent position
      d.   all of the above

38. Which of the following signs are associated with a partial airway obstruction with poor air exchange?

    a. a weak ineffective cough
    b. stridor
    c. cyanosis
    d. all of the above

39. The correct position for a chest thrust, while treating an infant with a complete foreign body airway obstruction is:

    a. one fingerbreadth above the xiphoid
    b. one fingerbreadth below the nipple line
    c. the nipple line
    d. the upper half of the breast bone

40. When a conscious infant with a complete airway obstruction becomes unconscious, you should <u>first</u>:

    a. attempt to ventilate and observe for chest excursion
    b. perform a jaw lift, examine the airway and perform a finger sweep if you visualize a foreign body
    c. administer 4 back blows and 4 chest thrusts
    d. check for a brachial pulse to establish the need for cardiac compressions

41. The primary disease(s) affecting the lower airways in pediatric patients is (are):

    a. asthma
    b. bronchiolitis
    c. pneumonia
    d. all of the above

42. Asthmatic attacks in children can be triggered by:

    a. upper respiratory infections
    b. allergies
    c. medication withdrawal
    d. all of the above

43. Asthmatic children with difficult breathing who become sleepy and lie down should receive:

    a. positive pressure ventilation
    b. humidified oxygen
    c. nebulized oxygen
    d. oxygen via nasal catheter

44.    It is not unusual for pneumonia in children to result in complaints of
       _____ pain, due to irritation of the diaphragm

       a.    neck
       b.    abdominal
       c.    back
       d.    pressure like

45.    Anatomically, foreign bodies that enter the lower airway are more likely to
       enter the _____ mainstem bronchus because it offers the more direct
       pathway at the division of the trachea.

       a.    right
       b.    left

46.    As in the adult, the _____ is the preferred method for
       opening the airway of an infant and child.

       a.    jaw thrust
       b.    head tilt-chin lift
       c.    head tilt-neck lift
       d.    chin pull

47.    While performing the maneuver described above, the head should be placed
       in the _____ position, to avoid kinking the membranous trachea.

       a.    hyperextended
       b.    extended
       c.    sniffing or neutral
       d.    slightly flexed

48.    When providing positive pressure ventilation in an infant, you should breathe
       at a rate of 1 breath every _____ seconds.

       a.    5
       b.    4
       c.    3
       d.    2

49.    While ventilating a patient with a bag-valve-mask resuscitator, if you note air
       leakage through the pop-off valve, you should:

       a.    use mouth
       b.    tape the valve closed
       c.    use a nonrebreather mask
       d.    do nothing and continue ventilating

50. When caring for a young drowning victim found in shallow water, you should automatically treat the child as if he had:

    a. kidney damage
    b. a cervical spine injury
    c. diabetes
    d. a bacterial infection

51. All of the following are considered risk factors of SIDS except:

    a. low socioeconomic group
    b. adolescent mother
    c. drug use during pregnancy
    d. postmature baby

52. SIDS is commonly confused with _____ by EMTs and police who respond:

    a. choking
    b. child abuse
    c. drowning
    d. overdose

53. A common cause of seizures in small children is:

    a. overdose
    b. fever
    c. aspiration
    d. vomiting

54. The most common internal organ injured in children is the:

    a. heart
    b. lungs
    c. spleen
    d. liver

55. The leading cause of death in children aged 1 to 14 years is:

    a. SIDS
    b. drowning
    c. accidents
    d. airway obstruction

## Chapter 14

### Case Histories

| Case History #1 |
| --- |

You respond to a call and find an alert 2 year old boy who appears to be in severe respiratory distress. Upon physical exam you note a barking cough, nasal flaring, intercostal retractions and stridor. The mother tells you that he had a recent upper respiratory infection and woke up during the night with difficulty breathing.

56. Based on the history and signs and symptoms, you strongly suspect:

    a.   asthma
    b.   epiglottis
    c.   croup
    d.   airway obstruction

57. The most important prehospital treatment of this patient is:

    a.   administering humidified oxygen
    b.   administering positive pressure ventilation
    c.   suctioning the airway
    d.   placing in the head down position

58. If this patient were to become completely obstructed, you should do all of the following except:

    a.   perform abdominal thrusts
    b.   attempted forced ventilation
    c.   rapidly transport to the hospital
    d.   place the head in the sniffing position

| Case History #2 |
| --- |

A 6 year old was struck by an automobile and thrown 10 feet. He is lying supine and is responsive to painful but not verbal stimuli. There is delayed capillary refill, and his skin is pale, cool and sweaty. The vital signs are pulse 150 and thready, blood pressure 60/40 and respirations 34 and shallow. There is no accessory muscle use or distended neck veins. Breath sounds are equal bilaterally.

59. Based on your assessment you suspect all of the following except:

    a.   hypovolemic shock
    b.   tension pneumothorax
    c.   cervical spine injury
    d.   internal bleeding

60.    Management of this child should include:

    a.    oxygen via nonrebreather mask
    b.    bag-valve-mask ventilation
    c.    ventilation with a manually triggered resuscitator
    d.    humidified oxygen via facemask

61.    Based on the vital signs you would suspect blood loss around:

    a.    10%
    b.    15%
    c.    20%
    d.    40%

62.    PASG is:

    a.    contraindicated
    b.    indicated
    c.    indicated only if the blood pressure drops to 50 systolic
    d.    applied but not inflated at this time

---

### Case History #3

You discover a 10 month old child in cardiopulmonary arrest with mottling of the skin in the dependent areas of the body and what appears to be black and blue marks around the torso. The parents said they put her to bed an hour ago and found her like this when they checked on her 10 minutes prior to your arrival. They say she had a recent upper respiratory infection.

---

63.    This child's condition has most likely been caused by:

    a.    abuse
    b.    choking
    c.    SIDS
    d.    heart failure

64.    Your action should be to:

    a.    wait for the police to arrive since the child is irreversibly dead
    b.    perform CPR and transport the baby to the hospital
    c.    not touch or move the baby in order to preserve evidence
    d.    record the parents statements very carefully and give them to the police upon arrival

---

### Case History #4

You respond to a 3 year girl with high fever, a sore throat, difficulty in swallowing and inspiratory stridor. She is sitting upright and leaning forward with her weight distributed on her hands, her mouth open, her tongue protruding and her chin thrust forward. She is very restlessness and drooling, and has a flushed face. Her breath sounds are diminished, but no wheezes or rhonchi are present.

---

65. Based on the history and signs and symptoms, you strongly suspect:

    a. bronchiolitis
    b. epiglottis
    c. croup
    d. asthma

66. The most important immediate action is:

    a. administering humidified oxygen
    b. examining the lower airway
    c. suctioning the lower airway
    d. placing the baby in the supine position

67. If this patient were to become completely obstructed, you should:

    a. perform abdominal thrusts
    b. attempt forced ventilations
    c. perform a finger sweep
    d. perform back blows

---

### Case History #5

You respond to a 11 month old girl who developed acute respiratory distress while playing with her toys in her crib. She appears to be crying, but no sounds are emitted from her airway. The parents tell you she has had no illness up to this event. You physical exam reveals chest movements without air exchange at the mouth and nose. Her lips are cyanotic, but there are no other obvious physical signs.

---

68. Based on the history and signs and symptoms, you strongly suspect:

    a. foreign body obstruction
    b. anaphylaxis
    c. bronchiolitis
    d. sleep apnea

69.   The most important immediate action is:

      a.   administering humidified oxygen
      b.   examining the lower airway
      c.   suctioning the lower airway
      d.   administering 4 back blows and 4 chest thrusts

70.   You continue your efforts without success, and the baby becomes
      unconscious.  You should first:

      a.   examine the airway
      b.   administer positive pressure ventilation
      c.   perform chest thrusts
      d.   perform back blows

71.   Two minutes later you are able to effectively ventilate the patient but you
      note that there is no pulse.  You should position your fingers
      _____ and begin cardiac compressions.

      a.   one fingerbreadth above the nipple line
      b.   one fingerbreadth below the nipple line
      c.   directly at the nipple line
      d.   just above the xiphoid process

72.   The appropriate compression rate for this patient is:

      a.   60-80
      b.   80-100
      c.   100
      d.   120

Skill Performance Sheet

**Child Mouth to Mouth Breathing**

Student Name_____     Date_____

| Performance Standard | Performed | Failed |
|---|---|---|
| Open airway with appropriate maneuver (head tilt-chin lift or jaw thrust) | | |
| Assess breathing (look, listen and feel) | | |
| Seal mouth around the patient's mouth and pinch nose | | |
| Give two smooth breaths while observing chest rise (1-1.5 seconds per breath) | | |
| Take mouth away between breaths | | |
| Check carotid pulse (pulse is present) | | |
| Give one breath every 4 seconds | | |

Comments_____

_____

_____

_____

Instructor _____     Circle One:   Pass   Fail

Skill Performance Sheet

## Infant Mouth to Mouth and Nose Breathing

Student Name_____     Date_____

| Performance Standard | Performed | Failed |
|---|---|---|
| Open airway with appropriate maneuver (head tilt-chin lift or jaw thrust) | | |
| Assess breathing (look, listen and feel) | | |
| Seal mouth around the patient's mouth and nose | | |
| Give two smooth breaths while observing chest rise (1-1.5 seconds per breath) | | |
| Take mouth away between breaths | | |
| Check brachial pulse (pulse is present) | | |
| Give one breath every 3 seconds | | |

Comments_____

_____

_____

_____

Instructor _____     Circle One:   Pass   Fail

Skill Performance Sheet

**Child One-Rescuer CPR**

Student Name_____          Date_____

| Performance Standard | Performed | Failed |
|---|---|---|
| Open airway with appropriate maneuver (head tilt-chin lift or jaw thrust) | | |
| Assess breathing (look, listen and feel) | | |
| Seal mouth around the patient's mouth and pinch nose | | |
| Give two smooth breaths while observing chest rise (1-1.5 seconds per breath) | | |
| Take mouth away between breaths | | |
| Check carotid pulse (pulse is absent) | | |
| If no pulse, locate correct hand position (lower half of sternum) | | |
| Maintain vertical position and provide 5 compressions (80-100/min) with heel of one hand while continuing to maintain head tilt | | |
| Provide one ventilation | | |
| After 10 cycles of 5:1, give two ventilations and check the pulse | | |
| If no pulse, continue 5:1 cycle | | |

Comments_____

_____

_____

Instructor _____          Circle One:  Pass  Fail

Skill Performance Sheet

## Infant One-Rescuer CPR

Student Name_____          Date_____

| Performance Standard | Performed | Failed |
| --- | --- | --- |
| Open airway with appropriate maneuver (head tilt-chin lift or jaw thrust) | | |
| Assess breathing (look, listen and feel) | | |
| Seal mouth around the patient's mouth and nose | | |
| Give two smooth breaths while observing chest rise (1-1.5 seconds per breath) | | |
| Take mouth away between breaths | | |
| Check brachial pulse (pulse absent) | | |
| Locate correct finger position (one fingerbreadth below the nipple line) | | |
| Maintain head tilt | | |
| Provide compressions at a rate of 100/per min (1/2 to 1 inch) with tips of fingers | | |
| Perform 10 cycles at 5:1 ratio | | |
| Check pulse | | |
| If no pulse, continue CPR | | |

Comments_____

_____

_____

Instructor _____          Circle One:  Pass  Fail

Skill Performance Sheet

**Complete Airway Obstruction in a Conscious Child**

Student Name_____          Date_____

| Performance Standard | Performed | Failed |
| --- | --- | --- |
| Confirm obstruction by asking "Are you choking?" | | |
| Apply manual abdominal thrusts | | |
| Repeat thrusts until effective or until the patient becomes unconscious | | |

Comments_____

_____

_____

_____

Instructor _____          Circle One:   Pass   Fail

Skill Performance Sheet

## Complete Airway Obstruction in a Conscious Child That Becomes Unconscious

Student Name_____          Date_____

| Performance Standard | Performed | Failed |
|---|---|---|
| Perform finger sweep (only if object is visible) | | |
| Open airway and attempt to ventilate | | |
| Apply 6 to 10 abdominal thrusts | | |
| Perform finger sweep (only if object is visible) | | |
| Attempt to ventilate | | |
| Repeat sequence of thrusts, finger sweeps and ventilation until effective | | |

Comments_____

_____

_____

_____

Instructor _____          Circle One:  Pass  Fail

# Chapter 14

## Skill Performance Sheet

## Complete Airway Obstruction in an Unconscious Child

Student Name_____     Date_____

| Performance Standard | Performed | Failed |
|---|---|---|
| Check for unresponsiveness | | |
| Position the patient supine | | |
| Open airway | | |
| Attempt to ventilate (obstructed) | | |
| Open airway and reattempt ventilation (obstructed) | | |
| Perform 6 to 10 abdominal thrusts | | |
| Perform finger sweep (only if object is visible) | | |
| Attempt to ventilate | | |
| Repeat sequence of thrusts, sweeps and ventilation until effective | | |

Comments_____

_____

_____

_____

Instructor _____     Circle One:  Pass  Fail

*Pediatric Emergencies*

Skill Performance Sheet

## Complete Airway Obstruction in a Conscious Infant

Student Name_____          Date_____

| Performance Standard | Performed | Failed |
|---|---|---|
| Confirm obstruction by observing infant (consider infectious cause of obstruction) | | |
| Perform four back blows | | |
| Perform four chest thrusts (same position as chest compression but at slower rate) | | |
| Repeat sequence of back blows and chest thrusts until effective or until the infant becomes unconscious | | |

Comments_____

_____

_____

_____

Instructor _____          Circle One:   Pass   Fail

Skill Performance Sheet

**Complete Airway Obstruction in a Conscious Infant That Becomes Unconscious**

Student Name_____                    Date_____

| Performance Standard | Performed | Failed |
|---|---|---|
| View airway and perform finger sweep (only if object is visible) | | |
| Open airway and attempt to ventilate (obstructed) | | |
| Perform four back blows | | |
| Perform four chests trusts | | |
| View airway and perform finger sweep (only if object is visible) | | |
| Open airway and attempt to ventilate | | |
| Repeat sequence of back blows, thrusts and ventilation until effective | | |

Comments_____

_____

_____

_____

Instructor _____        Circle One:   Pass   Fail

Skill Performance Sheet

## Complete Airway Obstruction in an Unconscious Infant

Student Name_____          Date_____

| Performance Standard | Performed | Failed |
|---|---|---|
| Check for unresponsiveness | | |
| Position the patient supine | | |
| Open airway | | |
| Attempt to ventilate (obstructed) | | |
| Open airway and reattempt ventilation (obstructed) | | |
| Perform four back blows | | |
| Perform four chest thrusts | | |
| View airway and perform finger sweep (only if object is visible) | | |
| Open airway and attempt to ventilate | | |
| Repeat sequence of back blows, thrusts and ventilation until effective | | |

Comments_____

_____

_____

_____

Instructor _____          Circle One:   Pass   Fail

## Chapter 15

## PSYCHOLOGICAL ASPECTS OF EMERGENCY CARE

Indicate which of the following methods of communication are effective versus not effective.

| Column A | Column B |
|---|---|
| *a* 1. focus your attention at the patient | a. effective |
| *b* 2. deal with the family not the patient | b. not effective |
| *A* 3. tell the truth | |
| *b* 4. never explain treatments-- it will frighten the patient | |
| *b* 5. never use the patient's name rather, refer to them as mom or dear | |

6. Which of the following age groups is most likely to commit suicide?

   a. small children
   b. persons in their 20s
   c. middle aged persons
   d. elderly persons

7. When caring for a sick or injured <u>child</u> who is afraid to go in the ambulance, your best approach would be to:

   a. encourage the child to bring along a favorite toy, doll or blanket
   b. assure the child that no one will hurt him at the hospital
   c. talk only to the parents, and let them deal with the child
   d. have the parents drive separately; the child will see their fear and become even more upset

8. When caring for a deaf patient, you should always remember to:

   a. speak loudly
   b. look directly at the patient when you speak
   c. obtain the history from a family member
   d. never allow a deaf patient to refuse medical aid

9.    When caring for a patient who is blind, it is best to:

    a.    maintain physical contact with the patient
    b.    refrain from touching the patient
    c.    treat the patient like a sighted person
    d.    explain each procedure after you do it

10.    You have a confused and agitated patient in your ambulance who thinks that he is in church and that you are his son. Your best approach would be to:

    a.    quietly go along with what he is saying or he will become more agitated
    b.    tell him that you are an EMT and that he is in an ambulance on the way to a hospital
    c.    let him think you are his son, but tell him where he is
    d.    restrain the patient and do not try to talk to him

11.    An emotional response to sudden illness, a death in the family or some other difficult personal experience that may be exhibited by anxiety, fear, paranoia, anger, hysteria, denial or withdrawal is called a:

    a.    situational reaction
    b.    nervous breakdown
    c.    hysterical reaction
    d.    temporary breach

12.    Nervousness, tension, pacing, hand wringing, and trembling are all symptoms of:

    a.    anxiety
    b.    paranoia
    c.    hysteria
    d.    suicidal tendencies

13.    A patient who is afraid that you are trying to kill him with poison gas when you place an oxygen mask over his face is suffering from:

    a.    anxiety
    b.    confusion
    c.    paranoia
    d.    hysteria

14.    The patient who is crying uncontrollably and beating her fists repeatedly against a wall or throwing herself to the ground is suffering from:

    a.    denial
    b.    confusion
    c.    hysteria
    d.    withdrawal

15. The patient who is having a heart attack and does not want to go in the ambulance because he "just has a little chest pain" is experiencing:

    a. denial
    b. hysteria
    c. anxiety
    d. confusion

16. A patient who experiences difficulty sleeping, loss of appetite, loss of sex drive, inability to feel pleasure and hopelessness is likely to be suffering from:

    a. denial
    b. depression
    c. hysteria
    d. psychosis

17. A person who is about to commit suicide:

    a. always exhibits signs of depression
    b. never calls for help
    c. may appear very content and even happy
    d. is never a danger to others

18. Distorted perceptions of reality, with hallucinations and inappropriate responses to the environment, best describes a:

    a. phobia
    b. situational reaction
    c. psychosis
    d. hysterical reaction

19. Signs of impending violent behavior include:

    a. pressured speech
    b. angry voice
    c. pacing
    d. all of the above

20. The first priority when faced with an emotionally disturbed patient is to:

    a. restrain him or her immediately
    b. consider possible medical causes
    c. give sedation and then restrain
    d. get permission from the family to restrain

21.    The first priority with a potentially dangerous patient is:

      a.     self-protection
      b.     the patient's protection
      c.     the legal implications
      d.     restraining him or her

22.    A good strategy when encountering a child who is refusing oxygen is to:

      a.     have the parent hold him down and administer oxygen via a face mask
      b.     give him a choice such as a simple face mask or a nasal cannula
      c.     tell him it is a toy that he can wear to the hospital
      d.     be firm and insist on the required therapy

23.    Which of the following represents the best way of identifying an elderly patient named Janet Jones?

      a.     hello, dear, how are you?
      b.     hello, ma'am, how are you?
      c.     hello, Mrs. Jones, how are you?
      d.     hello, mom, how are you?

24.    A suicidal patient who is explaining her reasons for wanting to commit suicide should be managed by:

      a.     comparing her problems to others and therefore minimizing their severity
      b.     acknowledging her perspective and offering her help at the hospital
      c.     being firm and taking a "parental role" in your relationship with her
      d.     waiting for an opportunity and quickly restrain her with the assistance of the police

25.    In general, the best posture to assume when dealing with a violent patient is:

      a.     firm and authoritative
      b.     aggressive and self-assured
      c.     calm and reassuring
      d.     light-hearted and carefree

26.    Responses such as guilt, grief, anger, hysteria, denial, withdrawal, or physical reactions are common reactions to:

      a.     phobias
      b.     pain
      c.     organic illness
      d.     death

27. When the family wants to view the body of a deceased loved one, in general you should:

    a. encourage them to avoid it to prevent hysterical reactions
    b. tell them that they can view it at a later time
    c. allow them to view the body
    d. make them wait until the physician arrives

28. A simple approach that an EMT can exercise when faced with the death of a patient and associated feeling of guilt or depression is to:

    a. share feeling with a coworker or friend
    b. take a clinical approach to avoid such feelings
    c. reason it out through positive thinking
    d. relate to it as a natural part of life and go on

29. Major disasters such as the death of children in a fire may require a more organized response by EMTs to resolve negative feelings. This process is called a(n):

    a. debriefing
    b. encounter group
    c. catharsis
    d. exchange session

## Case Histories

| Case History #1 |
|---|
| You have a female patient who appears to have been badly beaten and possibly raped. She refuses to answer questions about where she is hurt or what happened to her. She simply stares into space and refuses to look at you. |

30. This patient's common reaction to a terrifying situation is known as:

    a. denial
    b. withdrawal
    c. confusion
    d. hysteria

31. Your first action in caring for this patient should be to:

    a. examine her to see if she was raped
    b. identify yourself in a gentle and reassuring manner
    c. focus on injuries not emotional issues
    d. have her describe the incident to experience an emotional catharsis

---

### Case History #2

You respond to a home and find a patient who is combative and angry. His family states that he is never like this and suddenly exhibited aggressive and dangerous behavior. The past medical history indicates no psychiatric disorders, but the patient has a history of heart disease, diabetes, chronic obstructive lung disease and a recently herniated spinal disc. The patient is taking inderal, insulin and valium. His color is normal and he is breathing adequately.

---

32.   This patient's condition is most likely related to:

   a.   psychosis
   b.   depression
   c.   hypoglycemia
   d.   a drug reaction

33.   Your action in caring for this patient should include:

   a.   administer a glucose solution
   b.   give epinephrine
   c.   restrain the patient using police and family
   d.   induce vomiting

---

### Case History #3

You are dispatched to a call for a patient with terminal cancer. At the scene, you encounter a 34 year old patient dying from leukemia. The patient is conscious and aware of his condition. He responds angrily to almost every request or comment made to him.

---

34.   This patient's reaction:

   a.   is very common with dying patients
   b.   suggests insensitivity on your part
   c.   must be dealt with firmly
   d.   should be actively converted by cheerfulness

35.   The most effective method for dealing with this patient is:

   a.   empathetic listening
   b.   firm interaction and directions
   c.   a detached clinical approach
   d.   distract him from his problems

| Case History #4 |
| --- |
| You are dispatched to a call for an emotionally disturbed patient. At the scene, you encounter a 78 year old male who is disoriented and experiencing hallucinations. He states that he sees ants crawling on his chest and abdomen and that they are eating him alive. |

36.     All of the following are possible explanations for this patient's behaviors <u>except:</u>

        a.     alcohol withdrawal
        b.     organic brain syndrome
        c.     LSD ingestion
        d.     depression

## Chapter 16

## LIFTING AND CARRYING PATIENTS

1. The scientific use of specific, predetermined methods of efficiently lifting large weights so as not to injure oneself is known as:

    a. body mechanics
    b. lift science
    c. lifting physics
    d. physiology of lifts

2. The largest bone in the body is the:

    a. skull
    b. tibia
    c. pelvis
    d. femur

3. When lifting a patient, you should use the muscles in your:

    a. lower back
    b. upper back
    c. legs
    d. pelvis

4. When lifting a stretcher, your body should be positioned:

    a. as close as possible to the stretcher
    b. as far away as possible from the stretcher
    c. at a 90 degree angle to the stretcher
    d. at a 45 degree angle to the stretcher

5. When carrying a stretcher, your abdominal muscles should be:

    a. tightened
    b. relaxed
    c. alternating between relaxed and tightened
    d. pushed outward

6. When carrying a stretcher, your back should be:

    a. flexed
    b. extended
    c. held straight
    d. slightly curved

7. A simple emergency one-rescuer evacuation technique in which the patient is pulled from a dangerous area by the shirt, sweater or jacket is called the:

   a.  sweater pull
   b.  torso drag
   c.  clothes drag
   d.  patient pull

8. An emergency evacuation technique where the rescuer assumes a low profile, wraps the arms of the patient around his or her neck and slides the patient along the floor is called the:

   a.  patient sweep
   b.  fireman's drag
   c.  smoke-free drag
   d.  low level pull

9. A rapid evacuation technique where the patient is carried over the shoulder of the rescuer and that can be used for patients who <u>do not</u> have suspected spinal injuries is called the:

   a.  shoulder sling
   b.  shoulder carry
   c.  fireman's carry
   d.  upright carry

10. When lifting a non-spinal injury patient from the floor to the chair or stretcher or when carrying a patient with two rescuers, the technique of choice is the:

   a.  log roll
   b.  blanket lift
   c.  extremity carry
   d.  direct carry

11. Which of the following devices is best suited for moving a patient over rough terrain?

   a.  wheeled cot stretcher
   b.  stair chair
   c.  Stokes basket
   d.  long spine board

12. When moving a wheeled cot stretcher along ground level, the _____ of the stretcher should move first.

   a.  head
   b.  foot
   c.  right side
   d.  left side

13. The most commonly used and effective method for placing a wheeled cot stretcher in the ambulance is the _____ method.

    a. side carry
    b. front and back carry
    c. sitting position
    d. vertical lift

14. In general, the cot stretcher is loaded into the ambulance head first. One exception to this is with _____, in which case loading should be feet first.

    a. a fractured extremity
    b. an obstetrical patient
    c. small children
    d. cardiac arrest

15. The first part to be fastened in a scoop stretcher is the:

    a. head section
    b. hip section
    c. foot section
    d. seat belts

16. An aluminum lifting device that splits in half to facilitate easy removal of a supine patient using shovel-like edges is called a:

    a. Stokes basket
    b. shovel stretcher
    c. scoop stretcher
    d. folding stretcher

17. The length of the scoop stretcher should be adjusted to a length longer than the patient:

    a. after the patient is secured to the stretcher
    b. when the loaded stretcher is on the ambulance
    c. before sliding the stretcher under the patient
    d. this is not an adjustable stretcher

18. The main function of a spine board, regardless of the design, is to:

    a. allow for stabilization of femur fractures
    b. make extrication from an MVA easier
    c. take up less room and be useful when there is more than one victim
    d. provide rigid support for the spinal column to prevent further injury

19. When performing a log roll, the EMT positioned at the patient's _____ should supervise the movements.

    a. head
    b. shoulder
    c. hip
    d. lower legs

20. Before lifting patients onto any spine board, you should always:

    a. give oxygen
    b. immobilize the cervical spine
    c. obtain a written consent
    d. ask the patient if he or she can turn the head to either side

21. The most commonly used technique for placing a supine or prone patient onto a long spine board is the:

    a. six man lift
    b. blanket drag
    c. two man lift
    d. log roll

22. When securing a patient to a long spine board, which of the following should be attached last?

    a. the leg straps
    b. the pelvic strap
    c. the head
    d. the chest strap

23. A stable patient in an automobile accident should be removed by a:

    a. rapid extrication procedure
    b. long spine board
    c. short spine board or Kendrick's Extrication Device (KED)
    d. scoop stretcher

24. In the rapid extrication procedure, the long spine board should be bridged to the car seat by:

    a. a rolling cot stretcher
    b. the back step of the ambulance
    c. the support of two bystanders
    d. the trauma kit

25. When using the rapid extrication procedure on the driver of a car, the EMT in the _____ changes position prior to the removal of the patient.

    a. front passenger seat
    b. driver's doorway
    c. back seat
    d. passenger doorway

26. When performing the rapid extrication procedure, the EMT who is supporting the _____ supervises the movements.

    a. chest and back
    b. legs
    c. cervical spine
    d. the stretcher

27. Once the cervical collar has been applied, the first movement used to position the patient for rapid extrication is to:

    a. rotate the legs 45 degrees toward the seat
    b. lower the patient to the board
    c. bend the patient forward
    d. slide the patient to the front of the seat

28. The standing takedown is commonly used for:

    a. drivers in automobile accidents
    b. ambulatory patients with suspected spinal injury
    c. patients on ledges
    d. combative patients

29. In the standing takedown, the EMT _____ supervises the movements.

    a. on the left side of the patient
    b. behind the board
    c. on the right side of the patient
    d. facing the patient

30. As the first step in the standing takedown, manual spinal immobilization should be performed:

    a. facing the patient
    b. on the side of the patient
    c. behind the patient
    d. on both sides of the patient

31.  When performing the standing takedown, the EMTs at the side support the patient:

     a.   at the elbow and chest
     b.   under the armpit and outer arm
     c.   at the chest and back
     d.   at the shoulder and hip regions

32.  In general, when performing the standing takedown, the EMT who is the _____ should be positioned behind the patient.

     a.   strongest
     b.   tallest
     c.   shortest
     d.   most senior

33.  When securing the straps of the short spine board, the _____ strap(s) should be attached last.

     a.   chest
     b.   leg
     c.   abdomen
     d.   head

34.  When moving or lifting a patient who is attached to a short spine board from a car to a stretcher, you should lift the:

     a.   board
     b.   patient
     c.   straps
     d.   clothing

35.  When performing the helmet removal, the head should be supported at the base of the occipital bone and at the:

     a.   temporal region
     b.   maxilla and orbital regions
     c.   lower margin of the mandible
     d.   frontal bone region

36.  When removing a helmet, the support of the occipital region is best described as:

     a.   none
     b.   slight support on the posterior side
     c.   lateral support of the bone
     d.   support of the full weight of the head

37.     When removing a helmet, the helmet is:

        a.      compressed medially
        b.      left neutral
        c.      spread laterally
        d.      rotated at a 90 degree angle

38.     When performing helmet removal on a helmet that has a face piece, the helmet may have to be rotated slightly to accommodate the:

        a.      frontal bone
        b.      nasal bone
        c.      maxilla
        d.      mandible

39.     When applying a Kendrick's Extrication Device (KED), the strap that should be tightened last is the _____ strap.

        a.      head
        b.      middle
        c.      lower
        d.      leg

40.     An excellent device for the removal of a patient on a mountain or hillside is the:

        a.      Stokes basket
        b.      Kendrick's Extrication Device (KED)
        c.      rolling cot stretcher
        d.      scoop stretcher

41.     The stair chair is best used for:

        a.      a conscious patient who can sit and who needs to be carried down narrow or steep stairs
        b.      an unconscious patient found injured on a flight of stairs
        c.      an active obstetrical patient
        d.      an extra patient in the ambulance when there are not enough stretchers

42.     Patients complaining of dyspnea are generally more comfortable transported in a _____ position.

        a.      semireclining or fully upright
        b.      prone
        c.      supine
        d.      left or right lateral recumbent

43. The unconscious medical patient who does not require resuscitation is generally placed in a _____ position to prevent aspiration in case the patient vomits.

    a. fully upright
    b. supine
    c. left lateral recumbent
    d. Kendrick's

44. Patients in need of resuscitation must be placed in the supine position on a:

    a. scoop stretcher
    b. spine board
    c. Stokes basket
    d. stair chair

45. Patients in acute abdominal distress will usually be more comfortable:

    a. if they are prone
    b. with their knees bent
    c. if they drink milk
    d. on a spine board

46. A conscious patient with an isolated head injury (in the absence of suspected spinal injury) should be transported in the _____ position.

    a. prone
    b. supine
    c. lateral recumbent
    d. semireclining

47. Medical patients who feel faint should be placed in the supine position with:

    a. the head turned to the side
    b. their legs elevated
    c. their head elevated
    d. their knees bent

48. Unstable hypotensive patients with multiple fractures of the lower extremities and suspected spinal injury should be fully immobilized with the:

    a. Hare traction splint
    b. long board splints
    c. long spine board and PASG
    d. Kendrick's Extrication Device (KED) and short board splints

49.     Pregnant trauma patients showing signs of hypovolemic shock (without suspected spinal injury) should be placed:

    a.    supine with legs elevated
    b.    in the left lateral recumbent position
    c.    in the prone position
    d.    in the semireclining position

50.     If a patient rescue requires lowering a patient with ropes along a hill or cliff, the device of choice is the:

    a.    scoop stretcher
    b.    long spine board
    c.    folding stretcher
    d.    Stokes basket

Match the problem in column B to the appropriate removal and/or transportation method in column A.

| Column A | Column B |
| --- | --- |
| A 51.  stair chair | a.  conscious chest pain in a five floor walkup |
| G 52.  sitting upright on a cot stretcher | |
| | b.  stable auto victim with suspected spine injury |
| C 53.  rapid extrication procedure | |
| E 54.  log roll onto long spine board | c.  unstable auto accident victim |
| B 55.  Kendrick's Extrication Device (KED) | d.  patient with abdominal pain |
| D 56.  supine on cot with legs flexed | e.  patient on street who was struck by a car |
| F 57.  left lateral recumbent position | |
| | f.  8 month pregnant patient with severe vaginal bleeding |
| | g.  patient complaining of dyspnea |

Skill Performance Sheet

## Long Spine Board Using a Log Roll Procedure

Student Name_____          Date_____

| Performance Standard | Performed | Failed |
|---|---|---|
| Team leader assumes in-line immobilization | | |
| Cervical collar is applied | | |
| Three rescuers are positioned on one side of patient (shoulder, pelvis, legs) | | |
| Spine board is positioned on opposite side of patient | | |
| On command from team leader, patient is rolled toward three rescuers | | |
| Board is slid under patient | | |
| On command from team leader, patient is rolled onto board | | |
| Patient is adjusted on board | | |
| Body then head is securely attached to spine board | | |

Comments_____

_____

_____

_____

Instructor _____          Circle One:  Pass  Fail

Skill Performance Sheet

**Rapid Extrication Procedure**

Student Name_____          Date_____

| Performance Standard | Performed | Failed |
|---|---|---|
| EMT #1 maintains cervical immobilization from behind the patient | | |
| EMT #2 performs primary survey and applies cervical collar | | |
| Car door is bent open as far as possible | | |
| EMT #2 takes over in-line from outside of the car | | |
| EMT #1 positions a spine board in the car on a cot stretcher and slides the end under the patient's buttocks | | |
| EMT #3 assumes a position on the other side of the seat from EMT #2 and supports the patients thighs | | |
| EMT #1 supports the patient's chest and back | | |
| On command from EMT #2, the patient is rotated at a 45 degree angle toward EMT #3 | | |
| On command, the patient is lowered down on the board | | |

CONTINUED ON NEXT PAGE

## Skill Performance Sheet

### Rapid Extrication Procedure (continued)

Student Name_____     Date_____

| Performance Standard | Performed | Failed |
|---|---|---|
| With EMT #1 supporting the axilla, EMT #2 maintaining in-line cervical immobilization and EMT #3 supporting the legs, the patient is slid up the board | | |
| The patient's torso is secured to the board | | |
| The patient's head and neck is secured to the board | | |
| The patient is secured to the stretcher | | |

Comments_____

_____

_____

_____

Instructor _____     Circle One:   Pass   Fail

Skill Performance Sheet

## Applying a Kendrick's Extrication Device (KED)

Student Name_____        Date_____

| Performance Standard | Performed | Failed |
|---|---|---|
| EMT #1 maintains in-line cervical immobilization from behind the patient | | |
| Cervical collar is applied | | |
| KED is positioned behind the patient | | |
| KED is pulled up securely in axillary region | | |
| Attach the chest straps | | |
| Attach the groin straps | | |
| Attached the head section | | |

(Adapted from the Prehospital Trauma Life Support Program)

Comments_____

_____

_____

_____

Instructor _____        Circle One:   Pass   Fail

Skill Performance Sheet

**Applying a Short Spine Board**

Student Name_____          Date_____

| Performance Standard | Performed | Failed |
|---|---|---|
| EMT #1 maintains in-line cervical immobilization from behind the patient | | |
| Cervical collar is applied | | |
| Board is positioned behind the patient | | |
| Attach the chest and groin straps placing pads to protect the patient | | |
| Secure head to board | | |
| Lift patient, not board, to long spine board | | |
| Release groin straps before lowering legs | | |

Comments_____

_____

_____

_____

Instructor _____          Circle One:  Pass  Fail

*Lifting and Moving Patients*

Skill Performance Sheet

**Performing a Rapid Takedown**

Student Name_____          Date_____

| Performance Standard | Performed | Failed |
|---|---|---|
| EMT #1 assumes immobilization from behind patient | | |
| A cervical collar is applied | | |
| EMTs #2 slides board behind patient | | |
| EMTs #2 and #3 stand on either side of the patient facing toward the board and slip their hands under the patient's axillary region and grasp the next highest opening on the board | | |
| EMTs #2 and #3 support the shoulder with their other hands | | |
| On command from EMT #1, the board is lowered smoothly to the floor | | |
| As the board is lowered, EMT #1 must allow the head to move slowly to the board | | |
| The patient's torso is secured to the board | | |
| The patient's head is secured to the board | | |

(Adapted from the New York State Health Department Critical Trauma Care Program)

Comments_____

_____

_____

Instructor _____          Circle One:   Pass   Fail

## Chapter 17

## DISASTERS AND TRIAGE

1.     Which of the following best represents a closed disaster?

    a.     a plane crash on a mountain with no access road
    b.     a building collapse in a city
    c.     a burning building
    d.     a multiple-car collision on a highway

2.     A predetermined response system with neighboring communities that ensures a large scale response of emergency vehicles during a disaster best describes a(n):

    a.     transfer agreement
    b.     mutual aid agreement
    c.     disaster plan
    d.     MCI strategy

3.     The sorting of casualties of war or other disaster to determine the priority of need and proper place of treatment best defines:

    a.     categorization
    b.     stacking
    c.     triage
    d.     designation

Match the condition in column B to the appropriate color triage tag in column A.

| Column A | | Column B | |
|---|---|---|---|
| 4. | red | a. | an unconscious patient with a head injury |
| 5. | yellow | | |
| | | b. | traumatic cardiac arrest |
| 6. | green | | |
| | | c. | multiple pelvic fractures |
| 7. | black | | |
| | | d. | fractured humerus |

8.     The secondary triage area is where treatment occurs and where:

    a.     patients are staged for transport
    b.     dead patients are packaged
    c.     the command post is ideally located
    d.     the communications center is established

9.  When a victim fears death, perceives limited escape and has no information about what happened, the likely outcome is:

    a.  suicide
    b.  depression
    c.  panic
    d.  psychosis

10. At the site of a disaster, drivers of emergency vehicles should:

    a.  participate in early triage and treatment
    b.  park as close to the accident as possible
    c.  remain with their vehicles
    d.  report to the triage officer

11. The rapid response of onlookers, rescuers and press at the scene of a disaster that results in the blockage of traffic routes is called:

    a.  accident crowding
    b.  convergence
    c.  focal obstruction
    d.  central merge

12. The process of demobilizing response vehicles and apparatus for the purposes of returning them to normal community service is called:

    a.  recovery
    b.  remobilization
    c.  reintroduction
    d.  rehabilitation

13. The rebuilding of the community in a physical and emotional sense after a disaster, a process that includes critical incident stress debriefing, is referred to as:

    a.  reconstruction
    b.  rehabilitation
    c.  recovery
    d.  restoration

14. The three EMS components of disaster management are:

    a.  command, triage and patient care
    b.  triage, patient care and transport
    c.  triage, communications and patient care
    d.  command, control and triage

15.  The log that records the patient distribution to ambulances and hospital destination is called the:

   a.   major event log
   b.   logistics sheet
   c.   transportation log
   d.   disposition log

16.  At a disaster scene, the person whose function is to control traffic flow, gather supplies, stage additional vehicles and communicate ambulance availability to the command post is the:

   a.   supply officer
   b.   transport officer
   c.   communication officer
   d.   triage officer

17.  The process by which participants are allowed to express their feelings about the incident and thereby relieve stress associated with the situation is called the:

   a.   catharsis
   b.   debriefing
   c.   critique
   d.   field exercise

## Case Histories

| Case History #1 |
| --- |
| You and your partner are the first to arrive at the scene of a large airplane crash in a hilly, wooded area. At least a hundred people were on the aircraft at the time of impact. The left wing of the plane is smoking. It is late fall at twilight, and it is starting to snow lightly, and the wind is blowing strong from the north. The nearest hospital is about 20 minutes away, but there is only a single small road to access the area, and several cars belonging to local residents are already beginning to block the road. Your partner is the driver. |

18.  This disaster can be described as

   a.   open, active
   b.   closed, active
   c.   open, contained
   d.   closed, contained

19. As you and your partner arrive at the disaster scene:

    a. your partner should stay with the ambulance while you do a scene survey
    b. radio for additional assistance, then both stay in the ambulance until at least one other vehicle arrives
    c. both should drive back down the road to block further traffic and radio for assistance
    d. radio for police, fire and rescue assistance, then both stay with the vehicle until firemen arrive

20. The driver of your vehicle will temporarily become the _____ officer.

    a. command
    b. triage
    c. traffic
    d. post

21. The best place for a temporary command post at this time would be:

    a. near the right wing of the plane
    b. 200 yards south of the plane
    c. 200 yards north of the plane
    d. in a building 1/2 mile away

22. Your partner discovers four injured patients: a 50 year old unconscious man with a head injury, a 16 year old boy in cardiac arrest, a 60 year old man with bilateral fractures of the radius and ulna, and a 35 year old man with an open fracture of the femur. Which patient should receive priority?

    a. 50 year old man
    b. 16 year old boy
    c. 35 year old man
    d. 60 year old man

23. The 16 year old described previously would be considered a _____ triage category.

    a. red
    b. yellow
    c. green
    d. black

---

### Case History #2

You respond to a city street where a hot dog vendor's propane tank has exploded, causing over 10 injuries.  The truck is engulfed in flames.  The scene is in absolute chaos, with people running in every direction screaming for help.

---

24.    This disaster can be described as:

    a.    open, active
    b.    closed, active
    c.    open, contained
    d.    closed, contained

25.    As you approach the disaster area, your first concern should be:

    a.    triaging and identifying the severely injured
    b.    calling for additional assistance
    c.    protecting yourself and bystanders
    d.    staying with the vehicle until firemen arrive

26.    Based on the conditions described, which service is likely to assume command?

    a.    EMS
    b.    fire
    c.    police
    d.    other agency

---

### Case History #3

Your discover four injured patients: a 25 year old man with 40% second and third degree burns, an unconscious 42 year old man with a open chest wound, an 18 year old woman with signs of hypovolemic shock, and a 58 year old woman with a fracture of the radius.

---

27.    Rank the these patients in order of priority treatment:

    1.    25 year old man
    2.    42 year old man
    3.    18 year old woman
    4.    58 year old woman

    a.    1, 3, 2, 4
    b.    2, 1, 3, 4
    c.    2, 3, 1, 4
    d.    1, 2, 3, 4

28.  The 18 year old described above would be considered a _____ triage category.

    a.     red
    b.     yellow
    c.     green
    d.     black

## Chapter 18

## EXTRICATION

1. The EMTs primary role at the automobile accident is:

   a. gaining access
   b. extrication
   c. disentanglement
   d. emergency care

2. The term used to describe an extrication that can be accomplished through the use of hand tools or skills such as opening locks is called:

   a. disentanglement
   b. light extrication
   c. strategic access
   d. rapid extrication

3. Because of the possibility of spilled gasoline at an automobile accident site, the least appropriate method of securing the scene is through the use of:

   a. reflectors
   b. flares
   c. road cones
   d. battery operated lights

4. Blocks of wood used to stabilize vehicles are commonly called:

   a. stacking blocks
   b. cribbing
   c. stabilizers
   d. construction blocks

5. When attempting to gain access through a window, the patient should be protected by:

   a. moving him or her away from the window
   b. tilting the car away from the patient
   c. covering the patient with a rescue blanket
   d. shattering the window from the inside out

6. When attempting to unlock a door equipped with a antitheft lock, an adjunct that is very helpful is:

   a. a washer
   b. a rigid metal rod
   c. a piece of thin rope
   d. motor oil

7.   To bend away the roof of an automobile, you must first:

   a.   cut completely through the rear posts
   b.   cut completely through the front posts
   c.   place a support structure inside the car
   d.   remove the rear windshield

8.   Which of the following is a useful device for creating a flap necessary to gain access to a door lock?

   a.   tire iron
   b.   crescent wrench
   c.   hacksaw
   d.   springloaded punch

9.   When creating a flap in a door to gain access to a door lock, the flap should be:

   a.   circular
   b.   oval
   c.   U shaped
   d.   square

10.   If access to the patient through the floor is absolutely necessary, the best access point can be identified:

   a.   by its relationship to the rear frame
   b.   as just in front of the gas tank
   c.   as alongside the drive shaft
   d.   by the drainage plug in the floor

11.   Upon gaining access to the interior of the car, you find a patient who is short of breath, pale, cool and sweaty, hypotensive, and who has a respiratory rate of 22. Your immediate reaction is to:

   a.   apply oxygen and a KED
   b.   rapidly extricate the patient
   c.   apply the PASG prior to extrication
   d.   begin positive pressure ventilation

12.   The fastest and best way to create a larger door opening is to:

   a.   remove the hinges and door
   b.   remove the inner door lining
   c.   cut through the roof
   d.   overbend the door outward

13. The simplest and best method for creating room between the driver and the steering wheel is to:

    a.      cut the steering wheel away
    b.      slide the seat back
    c.      distort the steering wheel
    d.      cut the steering wheel post off

14. If cutting through a steering wheel is necessary, the two tools needed to do the job are:

    a.      mastic knife and band saw
    b.      ax and pry bar
    c.      crescent wrench and hacksaw
    d.      blowtorch and bolt cutters

15. Two things needed to effectively disentangle a foot caught beneath a brake are:

    a.      pry bar and hacksaw
    b.      chain and car door
    c.      tire iron and jack
    d.      cribbing and tire iron

16. If cribbing is not available for stabilizing an overturned car, you can use the:

    a.      seat cushion
    b.      air filter cover
    c.      spare tire
    d.      back of the seat

17. One method of reducing the number of glass shards when breaking a car window is to:

    a.      wet the window
    b.      tape the corners
    c.      apply contact paper
    d.      heat the window

18. A hand-operated <u>pneumatic</u> device used to spread metal is called a:

    a.      come-a-long
    b.      winch
    c.      pry-all
    d.      porter power

19.　The process of sorting and categorizing casualties that is derived from the French word meaning "to sort" or "to choose" is called:

　　a.　triage
　　b.　prioritization
　　c.　labeling
　　d.　stacking

20.　The optimal time from injury to arrival at the operating room is sometimes referred to as the:

　　a.　prime time
　　b.　critical minutes
　　c.　magic minutes
　　d.　golden hour

21.　The placement of traffic cones primarily depends upon the:

　　a.　speed limit of the road where the accident occurred
　　b.　weather conditions at the time of the accident
　　c.　width of the road at the accident scene
　　d.　type of road surface at the accident scene

22.　The first cone or traffic delineation device at an accident scene should be placed at _____ times the average stopping distance of a vehicle on that roadway.

　　a.　1 1/2
　　b.　3
　　c.　5
　　d.　10

23.　If electrical wires are down at a scene, you should do all of the following except:

　　a.　retreat to a position of safety
　　b　establish a hazard zone
　　c.　advise the occupants not to exit
　　d.　rescue occupants with a rope

24.　A patient is accessed from the floor:

　　a.　as a last resort
　　b.　as a primary approach
　　c.　as a routine procedure
　　d.　only for removal

25. The first thing you should do when approaching an automobile accident scene is to:

   a.   immediately call a tow truck for assistance
   b.   call for additional units
   c.   perform a windshield survey
   d.   park your vehicle 500 feet from the accident

## Case Histories

| Case History #1 |
| --- |
| You respond to a call and find two cars in a head-on collision.  You note through the windshield that the passengers and driver of car #1 are ambulating and talking to bystanders.  The passenger from car #2 appears in severe distress and the driver appears to be dead. |

26. Your first action upon leaving the ambulance is to:

   a.   evaluate the passenger of car #2
   b.   call for three additional units
   c.   make sure the scene is safe
   d.   perform CPR on driver #2

27. Upon approaching car #2, you note that all of the doors are jammed, the windows are closed, and the passenger is too confused to cooperate in opening the door. You should gain access to the patient by:

   a.   breaking the windshield
   b.   cutting through the floor
   c.   cutting through the roof
   d.   breaking the rear driver-side window

28. After you have gained access and pried open the car door, you find the patient in severe respiratory distress, with paradoxical breathing, and pale, cool and sweaty skin. Your immediate action should be to:

   a.   apply PASG
   b.   apply a short spine board
   c.   rapidly extricate the patient
   d.   perform a secondary survey

---

### Case History #2

Upon arriving at the scene of a car accident, you encounter a car with flames coming from beneath the hood.  You note a driver and two passengers who are trapped in the car.

---

29.    Your immediate action should be to:

   a.    attempt to extinguish the fire
   b.    cut a flap in the door to gain access
   c.    break the front windshield to gain access
   d.    cut a roof flap to gain access

30.    By the time your patients are in the ambulance, you note that they are all dyspneic and have cherry red complexions. You suspect:

   a.    cyanide poisoning
   b.    first degree burns
   c.    carbon monoxide poisoning
   d.    hyperthermia

31.    The most important treatment for these patients is:

   a.    humidified oxygen via a Venturi mask
   b.    oxygen via a nonrebreather mask
   c.    nasal cannula oxygen
   d.    cool compresses to their faces

---

### Case History #3

You and your partner are the first to arrive at the scene of an accident where a single car has struck a pole and rolled over onto its side.  You hear a baby crying from inside the car.

---

32.    Your immediate action should be to:

   a.    gain access and evaluate the baby
   b.    place cribbing to stabilize the vehicle
   c.    call for additional rescue personnel
   d.    gently roll the car onto its tires

33. Access through the roof has what one major disadvantage in this instance?

    a. roof entry compromises the structural integrity of an overturned car
    b. patients in an overturned car are in poor position for removal through the roof
    c. an overturned car is more likely to catch fire, and roof cutting causes sparks
    d. roof removal takes longer than floor removal, which is the method of choice in this instance

---

### Case History #4

You respond to a call at a railroad yard and are told that two men have fallen inside a huge tanker. You climb to the top of the tanker and look down inside to see the two men approximately 15 feet below you. They do not respond when you call out to them.

---

34. Your immediate action should be to:

    a. enter the car with a nonrebreather mask on your face
    b. allow oxygen to flow through tubing to clear the environment, then enter
    c. lower your partner with a rope to allow for rapid removal
    d. contact a rescue unit with scuba equipment

## Chapter 19

## AMBULANCE OPERATIONS

1.      Although driving is considered a physical task, it is ___ % cerebral in nature.

        a.      50
        b.      60
        c.      70
        d.      90

2.      The superior braking technique when driving an ambulance is:

        a.      left foot braking
        b.      right foot braking
        c.      dominant foot braking
        d.      alternate foot braking

3.      Palming the wheel in a turn represents a:

        a.      poor driving habit
        b.      method of stable turning
        c.      method for "feeling" the turn
        d.      accident avoidance technique

4.      Exemptions of traffic regulations provided by law for persons driving emergency vehicle are best described as:

        a.      necessary evils
        b.      privileges
        c.      protections from accidents
        d.      legal protections

5.      The basic hand positions when driving an emergency vehicle are:

        a.      11:00 and 1:00 o'clock
        b.      10:00 and 2:00 o'clock
        c.      9:00 and 3:00 o'clock
        d.      8:00 and 4:00 o'clock

6.      The correct position of a lap belt is across the:

        a.      umbilicus
        b.      thigh
        c.      pelvic girdle
        d.      upper thigh

7. Being thrown clear of the accident:

   a. has a very low probability
   b. is a common event
   c. is a less serious mechanism of injury
   d. is a planned response to an accident

8. The chances of being injured by a seatbelt are approximately 1 out of _____ accidents.

   a. 5
   b. 10
   c. 50
   d. 200

9. Emergency lights and sirens:

   a. are necessary to relieve the operator of liability in case of an accident
   b. are most effective in low-light situations, such as at dawn or dusk
   c. do not relieve the operator of liability in the event of an accident
   d. are most effective at high speeds

10. The most effective colors for rear-facing warning lamps are:

    a. amber and blue
    b. red and white
    c. red and yellow
    D. yellow and white

11. Four-way hazard lights:

    a. should not be used in a moving vehicle
    b. should be turned off when the vehicle is parked
    c. are necessary in a moving ambulance
    d. are most effective in low-light situations

12. The most effective warning lights are mounted:

    a. just above the rear bumper
    b. on the roof
    c. at eye level to other drivers
    d. in the outermost corners of the vehicle

13. The sound pattern of a siren in a moving ambulance is best described as:

    a. a circle with the siren at the center
    b. a square with the siren at the center
    c. a cone ahead of the vehicle
    d. a straight line in front of the vehicle

14. At 60 mph, the sound emitted from an ambulance siren:

   a.   moves more quickly through the air
   b.   barely precedes the ambulance
   c.   is louder on the sides of the vehicle
   d.   will not be heard inside the ambulance

15. The sweaty palms, rapid pulse and tense muscles felt by the operator of an emergency vehicle when the siren is switched on can cause the operator to immediately begin speeding. This response is the result of:

   a.   endorphin release
   b.   adrenalin release
   c.   physical demands of driving
   d.   vagal stimulation

16. An escort vehicle should be used only when:

   a.   the ambulance is traveling at high speeds
   b.   the operator is unfamiliar with the route
   c.   police are available
   d.   there is more than one ambulance

17. The two major control tasks of an emergency vehicle operator are speed control and:

   a.   vehicle balance
   b.   braking
   c.   radio communications
   d.   directional control

18. Van ambulances with raised tops:

   a.   have decreased wind resistance
   b.   have a higher center of gravity
   c.   are more stable during turns
   d.   usually have steel roof skins

19. When suddenly braking an ambulance, the rear brakes:

   a.   are considerably less effective than the front
   b.   do most of the braking
   c.   brake equally with the front brakes
   d.   allow for better directional control

20. The physical force responsible for most rollover accidents during turns is:

   a.   inertia
   b.   centrifugal
   c.   momentum
   d.   resistance

21.   The potential for a rollover is greater when the bank of the turn is:

    a.   very flat
    b.   steep
    c.   downhill
    d.   uphill

22.   The vehicle weight and speed:

    a.   have no effect on the potential for rollover
    b.   increase the chance for a rollover if both are high
    c.   increase the chance for a rollover if both are low
    d.   increase the chance of a rollover as the speed increases and the weight decreases

23.   When rolling friction is lost, you lose all of the following except:

    a.   forward momentum
    b.   directional control
    c.   centrifugal force
    d.   stopping ability

24.   When the brakes lock, the wheels stop turning and:

    a.   centrifugal force is lost
    b.   the stopping distance is decreased
    c.   stopping friction is lost
    d.   momentum is lost

25.   The technique in which the brake pedal is depressed to the point that the brakes lock, then the pedal is let up slightly to release the lock and then "quivered" at this lockpoint for maximum braking potential without loss of friction:

    a.   is called threshold braking
    b.   is useful only with antilock brakes
    c.   causes loss of steering control
    d.   increases centrifugal force

26.   A good way to judge the correct traveling distance between your ambulance and the vehicle in front of you in dry weather is to observe the vehicle in front of you as it passes a fixed object (such as a telephone pole) and then be able to count _____ seconds before you reach the same object.

    a.   2
    b.   4
    c.   10
    d.   12

27.  On icy roads, the above rule is increased to:

　　　a.　6 seconds
　　　b.　12 seconds
　　　c.　20 seconds
　　　d.　30 seconds

28.  Most emergency vehicle accidents occur:

　　　a.　on highways
　　　b.　at the scene of the accident
　　　c.　en route to an accident
　　　d.　at intersections

29.  Which of the following represents the best "nonjudgmental" documentation of a suspected case of alcohol intoxication on an ambulance call report?

　　　a.　the patient appeared intoxicated with an alcohol-like compound
　　　b.　there was an alcohol-like smell on the patient's breath
　　　c.　the patient was speaking as if he were intoxicated
　　　d.　the patient was extremely intoxicated

30.  Body diagrams on an ambulance call report are a useful way to document:

　　　a.　wounds and areas of pain
　　　b.　the patient's sex
　　　c.　the height of the patient
　　　d.　the position that the patient was found in

31.  What is wrong with the documentation, "The patient has a possible fracture of the ileum"?

　　　a.　it is too conclusive in its observation
　　　b.　it is too vague in its observation
　　　c.　a spelling error has made it unclear
　　　d.　it lacks a verb and a noun

32.  Which of these statements is least effective when documenting biological death?

　　　a.　the patient was dead for 30 minutes prior to our arrival
　　　b.　the patient has extreme dependent lividity on the back and posterior legs
　　　c.　the patient has evidence of rigor mortis in all extremities
　　　d.　the patient has suffered severe destruction of the skull and brain from the fall

33. Three o'clock P.M. is expressed in military time as:

 a. 0300 hours
 b. 1300 hours
 c. 1500 hours
 d. 1700 hours

34. Midnight is expressed in military time as:

 a. 0000 hours
 b. 1200 hours
 c. 2400 hours
 d. 0100 hours

35. Directing a bystander over the phone on how to perform CPR is:

 a. a dangerous technique
 b. used in many systems
 c. against heart association standards
 d. too time-consuming

36. Which of the following is <u>least</u> effective as a witness to refusal of care?

 a. the patient's family member
 b. a bystander
 c. your partner
 d. a police officer

37. Which of the following is <u>most</u> effective as a witness to refusal of care?

 a. the patient's family member
 b. a bystander
 c. your partner
 d. a police officer

38. If a patient who is refusing care also refuses to sign a release form, you should:

 a. force the patient to go to the hospital
 b. have a witness document the refusal
 c. continue caring for the patient until he or she signs the form
 d. remain on the scene until the patient signs the form

39. The refusal signature is of no value unless you:

    a. inform the patient of the potential consequences of refusal
    b. have at least two copies of the refusal
    c. have a police officer as a witness to the refusal
    d. have rendered at least some first aid care

40. Ecchymosis in the most dependent areas of the body that occurs after death is called:

    a. rigor mortis
    b. dependent lividity
    c. ecchymortis
    d. death discoloration

41. Which of the following facts is appropriate for the EMT to release to the press without breaching patient confidentiality?

    a. the patient's name
    b. the location of the call
    c. the field diagnosis
    d. the statements made by the patient

42. When an EMT wants to know the availability of beds in a given hospital, the best procedure to follow is to:

    a. consult the dispatcher
    b. radio each hospital directly
    c. go to the closest hospital and ask
    d. know each hospital before you respond

43. The initials UHF stand for:

    a. uniformed hailing frequencies
    b. unlimited height frequencies
    c. ultrahigh frequencies
    d. universal handling frequencies

44. A receiver transmitter that is placed at strategic locations to boost the strength of a radio signal is called a(n):

    a. repeater system
    b. transmitter booster
    c. acceleration system
    d. strategic signal booster

45. The major disadvantage of a handheld portable radio versus the ambulance radio is:

   a.   the need to carry extra equipment
   b.   it has a shorter range
   c.   it is more difficult to operate
   d.   it comes only in simplex

46. The method by which biological data are transferred from one location to another via radio is:

   a.   bioscopy
   b.   biogram
   c.   biometrics
   d.   biotelemetry

47. A good rule to follow when speaking into a radio microphone is to:

   a.   talk more loudly than normal while holding the microphone right next to your mouth
   b.   speak in a normal voice with the microphone a few inches away from your mouth
   c.   speak more slowly than normal in a low voice
   d.   speak normally with the microphone touching your lower lip

Match the descriptions in column B to the ambulance type in column A.

| Column A | | Column B | |
| --- | --- | --- | --- |
| C 48. | type I | a. | van-type ambulance |
| A 49. | type II | b. | modular patient compartment with van chassis |
| B 50. | type III | | |
| | | c. | modular patient compartment with truck chassis |

51. If sterile supplies such as bandages or dressings become wet, they should be:

   a.   dried in an autoclave
   b.   air dried
   c.   discarded
   d.   dried under ultraviolet light

## Chapter 20

### APPROACH TO THE MULTIPLE-TRAUMA PATIENT

Match the category in column B with the appropriate injuries in column A. Column B items can be used more than once.

| Column A | | Column B | |
|---|---|---|---|
| *c* 1. | uncomplicated fracture | a. | category 1 (most severe) |
| A 2. | unstable chest injury | b. | category 2 |
| A 3. | penetrating abdominal wound | c. | category 3 (least severe |
| B 4. | multiple rib fractures without a flail chest | | |
| A 5. | multiple pelvic fractures | | |

6. In an injury from a gunshot wound, the <u>most important variable</u> in determining the extent of injury is the:

    a. weight of the bullet
    b. distance traveled by the bullet
    c. velocity of the bullet
    d. material the bullet is made of

7. The airway maneuver of choice for a patient with a suspected spinal injury is the:

    a. head tilt-chin lift
    b. head tilt-neck lift
    c. jaw thrust without head tilt
    d. triple airway maneuver

Match the mechanisms in column B with the injuries in column A.

| Column A | | Column B | |
|---|---|---|---|
| B 8. | liver split by ligamentum teres with resulting hemorrhage | a. | compression |
| | | b. | deceleration |
| C 9. | puncture of stomach and small and large intestines | c. | penetrating |
| A 10. | rupture of the diaphragm | | |

11. Which of the following fractures is commonly associated with a heel bone fracture?

    a. lumbar spine
    b. iliac crest
    c. metacarpal
    d. pubic rami

12. Which of the following injuries is most likely the result of a side collision in an auto accident?

    a. clavicle fracture
    b. sternum fracture
    c. whiplash injury
    d. posterior hip dislocation

13. When a group of four people are in a car that is involved in a left front end injury accident in which the car rotates around the point of impact, the most likely person to be severely injured is the:

    a. driver
    b. front seat passenger
    c. rear right passenger
    d. rear left passenger

14. The most common mechanism for upper extremity fractures is?

    a. dashboard injuries
    b. fall on an outstretched arm
    c. machine accidents
    d. assault

15. A dashboard injury is likely to result in which of the following injuries?

    a. femur fracture
    b. posterior hip dislocation
    c. patellar fracture
    d. all of the above

16. The need for positive pressure ventilation should be determined when the respiratory rate is below 12 and above:

    a. 18
    b. 20
    c. 24
    d. 30

17. Which of the following is <u>not</u> usually associated with a closed head injury in an adult?

    a. hypovolemic shock
    b. spinal cord injury
    c. increased intracranial pressure
    d. respiratory depression

18. Dyspnea, stridor, cyanosis and subcutaneous emphysema around the neck and upper chest are most likely related to:

    a. pericardial tamponade
    b. injury to the large airways
    c. tension pneumothorax
    d. cardiac contusion

19. Tracheal shift, distended neck veins and absent breath sounds on one side are most likely caused by a(n):

    a. pericardial tamponade
    b. injury to the large airways
    c. tension pneumothorax
    d. cardiac contusion

20. When encountering a serious multiple-trauma patient, the blood pressure can be estimated by the loss of pulses in central and peripheral arteries. Loss of the radial pulse implies a blood pressure below ____mmHg.

    a. 50
    b. 60
    c. 70
    d. 80

21. Capillary refill is considered delayed when the refill time (minimally) exceeds _____ second(s).

    a. 1
    b. 2
    c. 4
    d. 5

22. In the mnemonic AVPU, which is used to remember the evaluation of central nervous system function, the "P" stands for:

    a. pressure
    b. paresthesia
    c. pain
    d. paralysis

23.     A cervical collar:

   a.     is the most effective form of cervical immobilization
   b.     completely restricts lateral movement of the neck
   c.     does not constitute spinal immobilization by itself
   d.     is the last step in the rapid extrication process

24.     In the mnemonic AMPLE, used to remember the essentials of a trauma history, the letter "E" represents:

   a.     events preceding the injury
   b.     evaluation
   c.     environment
   d.     emphysema

25.     Battle's sign is suggestive of:

   a.     epidural hematoma
   b.     skull fracture
   c.     facial fracture
   d.     subarachnoid hemorrhage

26.     Abdominal rigidity:

   a.     has a rapid onset with abdominal hemorrhage in the abdominal cavity
   b.     may take hours to develop from bleeding in the abdominal cavity
   c.     is the first sign of bleeding within the abdominal cavity
   d.     is never associated with bleeding within the abdominal cavity

## Case Histories

| Case History #1 |
|---|
| You respond to a collision in which a car has struck a utility pole and the front end is compressed into the passenger compartment. The driver is lethargic and complaining of pain in his left chest and abdomen. Your physical exam reveals respirations 32 and shallow, pulse 40 and regular, and blood pressure 80/60. You note paradoxical chest wall movements on the left side. |

27. Based on this description, your immediate action would be to:

    a. rapidly extricate the patient
    b. lay the seat back and apply the PASG
    c. perform a secondary survey
    d. apply a KED and remove the patient

28. Based on the pulse rate and the mechanism of injury, what underlying chest injury do you suspect?

    a. pericardial tamponade
    b. cardiac contusion
    c. tension pneumothorax
    d. pulmonary embolus

29. What condition does the sign on the left chest wall suggest?

    a. hemothorax
    b. pneumohemothorax
    c. cardiac tamponade
    d. flail chest

30. Given the mental state, paradoxical breathing and the respiratory rate, what approach to oxygenation seems most appropriate at this time?

    a. oxygen via nonrebreather mask
    d. oxygen via nasal cannula
    c. oxygen via bag-valve-mask with reservoir
    c. oxygen via face mask at 8-10 L/min

---

### Case History #2

A passenger in the same car is a 32 year old friend of the patient just extricated. He states that he was thrown forward against the dashboard and is in respiratory distress. The vital signs are pulse 120 and thready, blood pressure 80/50, and respirations 28 and shallow. His trachea is deviated to the right, and he has distended neck veins and subcutaneous emphysema on the upper chest and about the neck. Breath sounds are decreased on the left as compared to the right chest.

---

31. Based on the presenting signs and symptoms, the most likely underlying condition in this patient is:

    a. tracheal injury
    b. flail chest
    c. tension pneumothorax
    d. pericardial tamponade

32. The distended neck veins are most likely related to:

    a. increased volume within the vessels
    b. obstruction of venous return
    c. heart failure
    d. vasodilation of the veins

33. The immediate advanced life support measure needed to stabilize this patient is:

    a. cricothyroidotomy
    b. tracheostomy
    c. needle decompression of the chest
    d. open chest massage of the heart

34. The prehospital treatment of this patient would include all of the following except:

    a. high concentration oxygen
    b. rapid transport
    c. spinal immobilization
    d. splint the chest wall

35. The deviated trachea in this patient is related to:

    a. increased pressure in the left chest cavity
    b. increased pressure in the right chest cavity
    c. increased pressure in the mediastinum
    d. tracheal injury and hemorrhage in the neck

| Case History #3 |
| --- |
| You respond to a call for a man shot and find a 20 year old man with a stab wound in the left anterior chest, 5th intercostal space.  He is lethargic, and you note pale, cool and sweaty skin, distended neck veins and normal breath sounds. His vital signs are pulse 140 and thready, blood pressure 80/60, and respirations 28 and shallow. |

36. Based on the mechanism of injury and the physical signs, what condition is most likely the cause of his problems?

    a. tension pneumothorax
    b. tear in the aorta
    c. cardiac contusion
    d. pericardial tamponade

37.     The treatment of this patient would include:

      1.      high concentration oxygen
      2.      oxygen via nasal cannula
      3.      rapid transport
      4.      supine position

      a.      1 and 4 only
      b.      1 and 3 only
      c.      2 and 3 only
      d.      1, 3 and 4 only

---

### Case History #4

You respond to a call for a pool injury. At the scene, you find an 18 year old male lying supine at the edge of the indoor pool. The patient is responsive to pain <u>only above the level of the clavicle</u> and appears pale, cool and sweaty. Bystanders state that he was drinking and dived into a shallow part of the pool and did not come up for about 2-3 minutes. The vital signs are pulse 80 and thready, blood pressure 80/60, and respirations 28 and regular. On physical examination, the patient is cyanotic around the lips, there is no movement of his chest wall during breathing (only his abdominal wall), and rales are auscultated bilaterally.

---

38.     Based of the finding, you suspect a spinal injury at the level of the:

      a.      lumbar vertebrae
      b.      thoracic vertebrae
      c.      cervical vertebrae
      d.      sacral vertebrae

39.     The "abdominal breathing only" suggests loss of:

      a.      diaphragm function
      b.      abdominal muscle function
      c.      intercostal muscle function
      d.      brain function

40.     The shock that this patient is experiencing is _____ in nature.

      a.      hypovolemic
      b.      vasodilatory
      c.      cardiogenic
      d.      obstructive

41.    The cyanosis is most likely related to:

      a.      chlorine poisoning and poor circulation
      b.      pulmonary edema and ventilation impairment
      c.      cyanide poisoning and shunting
      d.      upper airway obstruction

---

### Case History #5

A 23 year old female passenger of a front end collision presents with the following: pale, cool and sweaty skin; contusion and tenderness in the upper left abdominal quadrant, and left shoulder pain. The left leg is flexed at the thigh, internally rotated and adducted. Her vital signs are pulse 130 and regular, blood pressure 110/80, and respirations 20 and shallow. You also note delayed capillary refill.

---

42.    Based on the presentation, you suspect a:

      a.      tear in the liver
      b.      stomach rupture
      c.      duodenum injury
      d.      ruptured spleen

43.    Based on the signs and symptoms, you estimate the blood loss at approximately:

      a.      less than 15%
      b.      15-30%
      c.      40-50%
      d.      greater than 50%

44.    The most likely extremity injury in this patient is a(n):

      a.      fractured of the pelvis
      b.      fractured shaft of the femur
      c.      posterior dislocation of the hip
      d.      anterior dislocation of the hip

45.    The shoulder pain is a good example of _____ pain.

      a.      radiation of
      b.      rebound
      c.      referred
      d.      visceral

46.    The early type shock that this patient is suffering from is classified as:

    a.    hypovolemic
    b.    obstructive
    c.    distributive
    d.    cardiogenic

---

### Case History #6

You arrive at the scene of a pedestrian struck by an auto and you find a patient who is responsive to pain by opening his eyes, moaning and flexing his arms. Bystanders state that he was thrown 20 feet and hit his head against the curb. He immediately lost consciousness, regained consciousness 5 minutes later and lost consciousness 10 minutes later (2 minutes before your arrival). You note a large hematoma on the right side of his forehead. His vital signs are pulse 42 and regular, blood pressure 200/120, and respirations 8 and irregular.

---

47.    Based on the history and physical assessment, you suspect:

    a.    hypovolemic shock
    b.    concussion
    c.    epidural or subdural hematoma
    d.    a small contusion

48.    The Glasgow coma scale score for this patient is:

    a.    3
    b.    7
    c.    9
    d.    12

49.    Based on the blood pressure and pulse, you suspect:

    a.    increased intracranial pressure
    b.    end stage hypovolemic shock
    c.    obstructive shock
    d.    distributive shock

---

### Case History #7

You arrive at the scene of a motor vehicle accident to find a conscious, agitated 28 year old male lying on the ground complaining of right thigh pain. He has a contusion over the anterior right thigh, and his right leg is rotated laterally. The blood pressure is 120/80, and his pulse is 100 and regular.

---

50.    Based on the signs and symptoms you suspect a:

      a.      fractured pelvis
      b.      fractured femur
      c.      posterior dislocation of the hip
      c.      fracture of the acetabulum

51.    The splint of choice for this patient is:

      a.      the long board splint
      b.      pillow splint
      c.      traction splint
      d.      tying the legs together

52.    The best pulse to evaluate circulation to the extremity in this injury is the:

      a.      radial
      b.      femoral
      c.      brachial
      d.      posterior tibial

EMT:PREHOSPITAL CARE

STUDY AND REVIEW GUIDE

ANSWERS

| CHAPTER 1 | | CHAPTER 2 | | | | | |
|---|---|---|---|---|---|---|---|
| 1. | A | 1. | B | 51. | D | 10. | H |
| 2. | C | 2. | E | 52. | A | 11. | E |
| 3. | C | 3. | F | 53. | C | 12. | K |
| 4. | D | 4. | A | 54. | B | 13. | B |
| 5. | B | 5. | C | 55. | C | 14. | B |
| 6. | B | 6. | D | 56. | B | 15. | A |
| 7. | C | 7. | A | 57. | D | 16. | A |
| 8. | C | 8. | A | 58. | A | 17. | C |
| 9. | A | 9. | C | 59. | D | 18. | D |
| 10. | A | 10. | C | 60. | C | 19. | B |
| 11. | C | 11. | C | 61. | B | 20. | D |
| 12. | C | 12. | A | 62. | A | 21. | B |
| 13. | D | 13. | E | 63. | C | 22. | D |
| 14. | B | 14. | B | 64. | D | 23. | B |
| 15. | D | 15. | D | 65. | A | 24. | A |
| 16. | A | 16. | B | 66. | C | 25. | D |
| 17. | C | 17. | C | 67. | D | 26. | C |
| 18. | D | 18. | A | 68. | A | 27. | A |
| 19. | A | 19. | C | 69. | B | 28. | C |
| 20. | B | 20. | B | 70. | D | 29. | C |
| 21. | F | 21. | D | 71. | D | 30. | B |
| 22. | A | 22. | B | 72. | D | 31. | B |
| 23. | D | 23. | D | 73. | A | 32. | A |
| 24. | E | 24. | A | 74. | D | 33. | C |
| 25. | D | 25. | A | 75. | C | 34. | B |
| 26. | D | 26. | B | 76. | D | 35. | A |
| 27. | D | 27. | C | 77. | B | 36. | A |
| 28. | B | 28. | D | 78. | A | 37. | B |
| 29. | A | 29. | D | 79. | B | 38. | C |
| 30. | B | 30. | C | 80. | B | 39. | C |
| 31. | A | 31. | C | 81. | B | 40. | C |
| 32. | A | 32. | C | 82. | A | 41. | A |
| 33. | B | 33. | B | 83. | C | 42. | B |
| 34. | C | 34. | A | 84. | A | 43. | C |
| 35. | C | 35. | B | 85. | B | 44. | C |
| 36. | B | 36. | A | 86. | C | 45. | A |
| 37. | A | 37. | D | 87. | B | 46. | A |
| 38. | D | 38. | C | 88. | C | 47. | D |
| 39. | C | 39. | C | 89. | C | 48. | B |
| 40. | B | 40. | B | 90. | A | 49. | D |
| 41. | D | 41. | A | | | 50. | D |
| 42. | B | 42. | D | CHAPTER 3 | | 51. | C |
| 43. | A | 43. | B | | | 52. | B |
| 44. | C | 44. | C | 1. | A | 53. | A |
| 45. | B | 45. | D | 2. | L | 54. | C |
| 46. | C | 46. | A | 3. | D | 55. | B |
| 47. | A | 47. | C | 4. | J | 56. | B |
| 48. | D | 48. | A | 5. | B | 57. | A |
| 49. | C | 49. | C | 6. | G | 58. | E |
| 50. | D | 50. | C | 7. | C | 59. | D |
| | | | | 8. | F | 60. | A |
| | | | | 9. | I | 61. | C |

**CHAPTER 3**

| | |
|---|---|
| 62. | B |
| 63. | D |
| 64. | C |
| 65. | D |
| 66. | C |
| 67. | C |
| 68. | C |
| 69. | C |
| 70. | D |
| 71. | A |
| 72. | D |
| 73. | B |
| 74. | C |
| 75. | B |
| 76. | B |
| 77. | D |
| 78. | B |
| 79. | A |
| 80. | B |
| 81. | B |
| 82. | B |
| 83. | C |
| 84. | A |
| 85. | D |
| 86. | A |
| 87. | B |
| 88. | B |
| 89. | B |
| 90. | C |
| 91. | A |
| 92. | B |
| 93. | A |
| 94. | C |
| 95. | D |
| 96. | A |
| 97. | A |
| 98. | B |
| 99. | D |
| 100. | C |
| 101. | C |
| 102. | B |
| 103. | D |
| 104. | B |
| 105. | A |
| 106. | B |
| 107. | B |
| 108. | A |
| 109. | C |
| 110. | C |

**CHAPTER 4**

| | |
|---|---|
| 1. | C |
| 2. | D |
| 3. | C |
| 4. | A |
| 5. | C |
| 6. | C |
| 7. | A |
| 8. | B |
| 9. | A |
| 10. | D |
| 11. | B |
| 12. | B |
| 13. | D |
| 14. | A |
| 15. | A |
| 16. | B |
| 17. | B |
| 18. | B |
| 19. | B |
| 20. | B |
| 21. | A |
| 22. | C |
| 23. | C |
| 24. | D |
| 25. | C |
| 26. | D |
| 27. | B |
| 28. | A |
| 29. | C |
| 30. | B |
| 31. | A |
| 32. | C |
| 33. | B |
| 34. | B |
| 35. | A |
| 36. | B |
| 37. | A |
| 38. | A |
| 39. | B |
| 40. | C |
| 41. | C |
| 42. | B |
| 43. | A |
| 44. | E |
| 45. | D |
| 46. | C |
| 47. | B |
| 48. | F |
| 49. | E |
| 50. | G |
| 51. | I |
| 52. | C |
| 53. | A |
| 54. | D |
| 55. | J |
| 56. | H |
| 57. | A |
| 58. | B |
| 59. | B |
| 60. | C |

**CHAPTER 5**

| | |
|---|---|
| 1. | B |
| 2. | B |
| 3. | C |
| 4. | C |
| 5. | D |
| 6. | A |
| 7. | A |
| 8. | D |
| 9. | D |
| 10. | B |
| 11. | D |
| 12. | C |
| 13. | D |
| 14. | B |
| 15. | D |
| 16. | A |
| 17. | C |
| 18. | A |
| 19. | C |
| 20. | A |
| 21. | D |
| 22. | C |
| 23. | C |
| 24. | A |
| 25. | A |
| 26. | B |
| 27. | A |
| 28. | C |
| 29. | D |
| 30. | C |
| 31. | B |
| 32. | B |
| 33. | B |
| 34. | B |
| 35. | A |
| 36. | B |
| 37. | C |
| 38. | B |
| 39. | D |
| 40. | B |
| 41. | C |
| 42. | D |
| 43. | B |
| 44. | B |
| 45. | B |
| 46. | B |
| 47. | A |
| 48. | C |
| 49. | A |
| 50. | B |
| 51. | A |
| 52. | B |
| 53. | A |
| 54. | A |
| 55. | C |
| 56. | A |
| 57. | A |
| 58. | C |
| 59. | C |
| 60. | C |
| 61. | C |
| 62. | D |
| 63. | C |
| 64. | B |
| 65. | C |
| 66. | D |
| 67. | C |
| 68. | A |
| 69. | B |
| 70. | B |
| 71. | A |
| 72. | C |
| 73. | D |
| 74. | A |
| 75. | D |
| 76. | B |
| 77. | D |
| 78. | B |
| 79. | B |
| 80. | B |
| 81. | C |
| 82. | A |
| 83. | D |
| 84. | C |
| 85. | D |
| 86. | B |
| 87. | B |
| 88. | D |
| 89. | B |
| 90. | B |
| 91. | A |

## CHAPTER 5

| | |
|---|---|
| 92. | B |
| 93. | D |
| 94. | D |
| 95. | B |
| 96. | C |
| 97. | C |
| 98. | D |

## CHAPTER 6

| | |
|---|---|
| 1. | A |
| 2. | A |
| 3. | C |
| 4. | B |
| 5. | C |
| 6. | C |
| 7. | A |
| 8. | A |
| 9. | B |
| 10. | C |
| 11. | C |
| 12. | D |
| 13. | D |
| 14. | B |
| 15. | D |
| 16. | C |
| 17. | A |
| 18. | A |
| 19. | C |
| 20. | A |
| 21. | C |
| 22. | C |
| 23. | A |
| 24. | B |
| 25. | A |
| 26. | C |
| 27. | B |
| 28. | B |
| 29. | C |
| 30. | B |
| 31. | B |
| 32. | A |
| 33. | B |
| 34. | A |
| 35. | C |
| 36. | B |
| 37. | B |
| 38. | B |
| 39. | C |
| 40. | B |

| | |
|---|---|
| 41. | C |
| 42. | A |
| 43. | B |
| 44. | B |
| 45. | A |
| 46. | C |
| 47. | D |
| 48. | B |
| 49. | A |
| 50. | B |
| 51. | A |
| 52. | B |
| 53. | A |
| 54. | B |
| 55. | B |
| 56. | A |
| 57. | D |
| 58. | C |
| 59. | C |
| 60. | D |
| 61. | D |
| 62. | C |
| 63. | D |
| 64. | A |
| 65. | C |
| 66. | B |
| 67. | A |
| 68. | D |
| 69. | A |
| 70. | B |
| 71. | B |
| 72. | C |
| 73. | C |
| 74. | B |
| 75. | D |
| 76. | C |
| 77. | A |
| 78. | A |
| 79. | D |
| 80. | B |
| 81. | B |
| 82. | C |
| 83. | A |
| 84. | B |
| 85. | E |
| 86. | C |
| 87. | C |
| 88. | A |
| 89. | D |
| 90. | C |
| 91. | A |
| 92. | C |

| | |
|---|---|
| 93. | C |
| 94. | C |
| 95. | C |
| 96. | A |

## CHAPTER 7

| | |
|---|---|
| 1. | A |
| 2. | G |
| 3. | H |
| 4. | C |
| 5. | D |
| 6. | F |
| 7. | E |
| 8. | B |
| 9. | A |
| 10. | D |
| 11. | B |
| 12. | D |
| 13. | A |
| 14. | C |
| 15. | B |
| 16. | A |
| 17. | D |
| 18. | A |
| 19. | B |
| 20. | A |
| 21. | B |
| 22. | A |
| 23. | A |
| 24. | B |
| 25. | B |
| 26. | B |
| 27. | E |
| 28. | A |
| 29. | B |
| 30. | D |
| 31. | C |
| 32. | A |
| 33. | D |
| 34. | C |
| 35. | B |
| 36. | A |
| 37. | A |
| 38. | B |
| 39. | C |
| 40. | A |
| 41. | B |
| 42. | C |
| 43. | D |
| 44. | B |
| 45. | D |

| | |
|---|---|
| 46. | A |
| 47. | C |
| 48. | E |
| 49. | C |
| 50. | A |
| 51. | A |
| 52. | C |
| 53. | C |
| 54. | A |
| 55. | D |
| 56. | B |
| 57. | B |
| 58. | C |
| 59. | B |
| 60. | C |
| 61. | A |
| 62. | A |
| 63. | C |
| 64. | B |
| 65. | C |
| 66. | C |
| 67. | B |
| 68. | B |
| 69. | B |
| 70. | B |
| 71. | C |
| 72. | A |
| 73. | D |
| 74. | C |
| 75. | A |
| 76. | B |
| 77. | B |
| 78. | B |
| 79. | A |
| 80. | B |
| 81. | C |
| 82. | B |
| 83. | A |
| 84. | B |
| 85. | B |
| 86. | C |
| 87. | B |
| 88. | A |
| 89. | B |
| 90. | A |
| 91. | C |
| 92. | C |
| 93. | B |
| 94. | C |
| 95. | A |
| 96. | A |
| 97. | C |

| | | | | | | | |
|---|---|---|---|---|---|---|---|
| 98. | B | 148. | C | 49. | C | 7. | B |
| 99. | B | | | 50. | A | 8. | E |
| 100. | D | **CHAPTER 8** | | 51. | B | 9. | C |
| 101. | D | | | 52. | C | 10. | D |
| 102. | C | 1. | G | 53. | E | 11. | A |
| 103. | B | 2. | J | 54. | D | 12. | B |
| 104. | A | 3. | E | 55. | A | 13. | A |
| 105. | B | 4. | F | 56. | B | 14. | B |
| 106. | B | 5. | I | 57. | C | 15. | B |
| 107. | A | 6. | D | 58. | C | 16. | B |
| 108. | C | 7. | A | 59. | A | 17. | C |
| 109. | C | 8. | K | 60. | B | 18. | A |
| 110. | B | 9. | C | 61. | B | 19. | D |
| 111. | D | 10. | B | 62. | C | 20. | B |
| 112. | C | 11. | H | 63. | B | 21. | A |
| 113. | B | 12. | L | 64. | A | 22. | A |
| 114. | D | 13. | C | 65. | B | 23. | A |
| 115. | B | 14. | C | 66. | D | 24. | D |
| 116. | B | 15. | C | 67. | B | 25. | C |
| 117. | C | 16. | C | 68. | C | 26. | A |
| 118. | A | 17. | D | 69. | C | 27. | D |
| 119. | A | 18. | B | 70. | C | 28. | B |
| 120. | A | 19. | B | 71. | A | 29. | C |
| 121. | A | 20. | B | 72. | B | 30. | C |
| 122. | B | 21. | B | 73. | A | 31. | C |
| 123. | D | 22. | C | 74. | C | 32. | A |
| 124. | B | 23. | A | 75. | B | 33. | B |
| 125. | C | 24. | B | 76. | A | 34. | A |
| 126. | A | 25. | C | 77. | A | 35. | B |
| 127. | C | 26. | D | 78. | B | 36. | C |
| 128. | C | 27. | D | 79. | D | 37. | A |
| 129. | A | 28. | B | 80. | B | 38. | B |
| 130. | D | 29. | B | 81. | C | 39. | D |
| 131. | B | 30. | B | 82. | A | 40. | B |
| 132. | B | 31. | B | 83. | C | 41. | A |
| 133. | A | 32. | A | 84. | B | 42. | B |
| 134. | D | 33. | C | 85. | B | 43. | C |
| 135. | A | 34. | A | 86. | B | 44. | B |
| 136. | B | 35. | D | 87. | A | 45. | B |
| 137. | D | 36. | D | 88. | D | 46. | A |
| 138. | A | 37. | A | 89. | B | 47. | C |
| 139. | B | 38. | D | 90. | C | 48. | B |
| 140. | A | 39. | D | 91. | A | 49. | A |
| 141. | A | 40. | C | | | 50. | A |
| 142. | B | 41. | A | **CHAPTER 9** | | 51. | C |
| 143. | C | 42. | A | | | 52. | D |
| 144. | B | 43. | C | 1. | C | 53. | A |
| 145. | B | 44. | C | 2. | A | 54. | C |
| 146. | A | 45. | D | 3. | C | 55. | C |
| 147. | B | 46. | A | 4. | D | 56. | A |
| | | 47. | A | 5. | C | 57. | B |
| | | 48. | C | 6. | A | 58. | B |

## CHAPTER 9

| | |
|---|---|
| 59. | C |
| 60. | B |
| 61. | A |
| 62. | C |
| 63. | B |
| 64. | B |
| 65. | C |
| 66. | D |
| 67. | A |
| 68. | B |
| 69. | D |
| 70. | C |
| 71. | B |
| 72. | A |
| 73. | C |
| 74. | B |
| 75. | C |
| 76. | B |
| 77. | A |

## CHAPTER 10

| | |
|---|---|
| 1. | A |
| 2. | C |
| 3. | A |
| 4. | B |
| 5. | C |
| 6. | D |
| 7. | A |
| 8. | B |
| 9. | H |
| 10. | A |
| 11. | B |
| 12. | G |
| 13. | E |
| 14. | C |
| 15. | D |
| 16. | F |
| 17. | C |
| 18. | C |
| 19. | A |
| 20. | C |
| 21. | B |
| 22. | A |
| 23. | B |
| 24. | C |
| 25. | D |
| 26. | A |
| 27. | E |
| 28. | A |
| 29. | G |
| 30. | H |
| 31. | I |
| 32. | C |
| 33. | F |
| 34. | D |
| 35. | B |
| 36. | A |
| 37. | C |
| 38. | C |
| 39. | C |
| 40. | A |
| 41. | B |
| 42. | C |
| 43. | A |
| 44. | B |
| 45. | B |
| 46. | C |
| 47. | C |
| 48. | F |
| 49. | E |
| 50. | B |
| 51. | D |
| 52. | A |
| 53. | D |
| 54. | B |
| 55. | C |
| 56. | B |
| 57. | C |
| 58. | A |
| 59. | C |
| 60. | C |
| 61. | D |
| 62. | A |
| 63. | B |
| 64. | D |
| 65. | C |
| 66. | C |
| 67. | C |
| 68. | E |
| 69. | F |
| 70. | B |
| 71. | D |
| 72. | A |
| 73. | A |
| 74. | C |
| 75. | B |
| 76. | B |
| 77. | C |
| 78. | A |
| 79. | B |
| 80. | B |
| 81. | A |
| 82. | C |
| 83. | B |
| 84. | B |
| 85. | A |
| 86. | C |
| 87. | B |
| 88. | B |
| 89. | A |
| 90. | C |
| 91. | A |
| 92. | B |
| 93. | D |
| 94. | B |
| 95. | B |
| 96. | D |
| 97. | C |
| 98. | C |
| 99. | A |
| 100. | A |
| 101. | B |
| 102. | A |
| 103. | B |
| 104. | B |
| 105. | C |
| 106. | B |
| 107. | A |
| 108. | C |

## CHAPTER 11

| | |
|---|---|
| 1. | A |
| 2. | D |
| 3. | B |
| 4. | C |
| 5. | A |
| 6. | D |
| 7. | C |
| 8. | C |
| 9. | A |
| 10. | B |
| 11. | D |
| 12. | B |
| 13. | B |
| 14. | B |
| 15. | A |
| 16. | B |
| 17. | C |
| 18. | D |
| 19. | E |
| 20. | B |
| 21. | D |
| 22. | A |
| 23. | A |
| 24. | A |
| 25. | C |
| 26. | B |
| 27. | A |
| 28. | D |
| 29. | B |
| 30. | C |
| 31. | A |
| 32. | A |
| 33. | C |
| 34. | C |
| 35. | C |
| 36. | A |
| 37. | B |
| 38. | B |
| 39. | C |
| 40. | A |
| 41. | C |
| 42. | B |
| 43. | A |
| 44. | C |
| 45. | D |
| 46. | C |
| 47. | A |
| 48. | B |
| 49. | C |
| 50. | D |
| 51. | A |
| 52. | A |
| 53. | B |
| 54. | C |
| 55. | B |
| 56. | A |
| 57. | B |
| 58. | A |
| 59. | A |
| 60. | B |
| 61. | C |
| 62. | C |
| 63. | B |
| 64. | B |
| 65. | C |
| 66. | B |
| 67. | B |
| 68. | C |
| 69. | A |
| 70. | D |
| 71. | E |
| 72. | F |
| 73. | C |

| CHAPTER 11 | | | | CHAPTER 12 | | | |
|---|---|---|---|---|---|---|---|
| 74. | A | 124. | A | 1. | A | 51. | B |
| 75. | A | 125. | C | 2. | C | 52. | C |
| 76. | 5 | 126. | B | 3. | C | 53. | A |
| 77. | 3 | 127. | A | 4. | C | 54. | A |
| 78. | 2 | 128. | A | 5. | B | 55. | B |
| 79. | 4 | 129. | B | 6. | D | 56. | B |
| 80. | 1 | 130. | D | 7. | D | 57. | C |
| 81. | B | 131. | A | 8. | A | 58. | C |
| 82. | B | 132. | B | 9. | D | 59. | B |
| 83. | D | 133. | C | 10. | D | 60. | B |
| 84. | C | 134. | B | 11. | B | 61. | C |
| 85. | C | 135. | A | 12. | D | 62. | C |
| 86. | C | 136. | C | 13. | B | 63. | A |
| 87. | C | 137. | A | 14. | B | 64. | A |
| 88. | C | 138. | B | 15. | B | 65. | C |
| 89. | B | 139. | A | 16. | A | 66. | B |
| 90. | B | 140. | B | 17. | A | 67. | C |
| 91. | D | 141. | A | 18. | B | 68. | B |
| 92. | A | 142. | B | 19. | B | 69. | D |
| 93. | C | 143. | C | 20. | A | 70. | D |
| 94. | B | 144. | B | 21. | B | 71. | C |
| 95. | E | 145. | C | 22. | B | 72. | C |
| 96. | B | 146. | D | 23. | B | 73. | D |
| 97. | A | 147. | A | 24. | D | 74. | A |
| 98. | C | 148. | C | 25. | B | 75. | C |
| 99. | A | 149. | A | 26. | B | 76. | B |
| 100. | C | 150. | A | 27. | A | 77. | D |
| 101. | B | 151. | A | 28. | A | 78. | C |
| 102. | D | 152. | B | 29. | D | 79. | C |
| 103. | C | 153. | D | 30. | A | 80. | C |
| 104. | A | 154. | B | 31. | C | 81. | A |
| 105. | D | 155. | C | 32. | C | 82. | C |
| 106. | C | 156. | B | 33. | B | 83. | B |
| 107. | B | 157. | C | 34. | D | 84. | C |
| 108. | B | 158. | B | 35. | B | 85. | C |
| 109. | B | 159. | B | 36. | A | 86. | A |
| 110. | B | 160. | A | 37. | C | 87. | D |
| 111. | D | 161. | C | 38. | C | 88. | B |
| 112. | A | 162. | B | 39. | C | 89. | B |
| 113. | C | 163. | C | 40. | B | 90. | D |
| 114. | A | 164. | A | 41. | A | 91. | B |
| 115. | B | 165. | C | 42. | A | 92. | C |
| 116. | C | 166. | A | 43. | D | 93. | A |
| 117. | C | 167. | B | 44. | B | 94. | C |
| 118. | A | 168. | B | 45. | D | 95. | B |
| 119. | B | 169. | C | 46. | B | 96. | C |
| 120. | D | 170. | B | 47. | B | 97. | B |
| 121. | B | 171. | A | 48. | A | 98. | B |
| 122. | B | 172. | A | 49. | C | 99. | D |
| 123. | B | 173. | B | 50. | B | 100. | D |
| | | | | | | 101. | D |
| | | | | | | 102. | C |

CHAPTER 12

| | |
|---|---|
| 103. | D |
| 104. | A |
| 105. | D |
| 106. | B |
| 107. | A |
| 108. | B |
| 109. | D |
| 110. | B |
| 111. | B |
| 112. | A |
| 113. | B |
| 114. | B |
| 115. | B |
| 116. | C |
| 117. | A |
| 118. | B |
| 119. | A |
| 120. | B |
| 121. | C |
| 122. | A |
| 123. | C |
| 124. | B |
| 125. | B |
| 126. | D |
| 127. | A |
| 128. | C |
| 129. | A |
| 130. | C |
| 131. | D |
| 132. | B |
| 133. | A |
| 134. | B |
| 135. | B |
| 136. | C |
| 137. | C |
| 138. | A |
| 139. | A |
| 140. | C |
| 141. | A |
| 142. | A |
| 143. | C |
| 144. | B |
| 145. | A |

CHAPTER 13

| | |
|---|---|
| 1. | C |
| 2. | H |
| 3. | E |
| 4. | F |
| 5. | A |
| 6. | B |
| 7. | G |
| 8. | D |
| 9. | D |
| 10. | F |
| 11. | E |
| 12. | C |
| 13. | G |
| 14. | B |
| 15. | A |
| 16. | B |
| 17. | D |
| 18. | A |
| 19. | C |
| 20. | B |
| 21. | B |
| 22. | B |
| 23. | B |
| 24. | B |
| 25. | B |
| 26. | D |
| 27. | C |
| 28. | D |
| 29. | A |
| 30. | B |
| 31. | B |
| 32. | C |
| 33. | C |
| 34. | B |
| 35. | B |
| 36. | C |
| 37. | B |
| 38. | B |
| 39. | D |
| 40. | B |
| 41. | C |
| 42. | B |
| 43. | B |
| 44. | A |
| 45. | B |
| 46. | D |
| 47. | B |
| 48. | B |
| 49. | B |
| 50. | C |
| 51. | C |
| 52. | D |
| 53. | D |
| 54. | A |
| 55. | A |
| 56. | D |
| 57. | C |
| 58. | D |
| 59. | B |
| 60. | C |
| 61. | C |
| 62. | B |
| 63. | A |
| 64. | C |
| 65. | B |
| 66. | C |
| 67. | A |
| 68. | D |
| 69. | C |
| 70. | B |
| 71. | B |
| 72. | B |
| 73. | B |
| 74. | B |
| 75. | C |
| 76. | B |
| 77. | A |
| 78. | C |
| 79. | D |
| 80. | B |
| 81. | B |
| 82. | A |
| 83. | A |
| 84. | B |
| 85. | B |
| 86. | B |

CHAPTER 14

| | |
|---|---|
| 1. | B |
| 2. | C |
| 3. | C |
| 4. | A |
| 5. | C |
| 6. | B |
| 7. | D |
| 8. | D |
| 9. | A |
| 10. | C |
| 11. | A |
| 12. | D |
| 13. | B |
| 14. | A |
| 15. | C |
| 16. | C |
| 17. | B |
| 18. | A |
| 19. | D |
| 20. | C |
| 21. | D |
| 22. | A |
| 23. | C |
| 24. | C |
| 25. | A |
| 26. | C |
| 27. | B |
| 28. | A |
| 29. | A |
| 30. | C |
| 31. | D |
| 32. | D |
| 33. | B |
| 34. | D |
| 35. | C |
| 36. | D |
| 37. | D |
| 38. | D |
| 39. | B |
| 40. | B |
| 41. | D |
| 42. | D |
| 43. | A |
| 44. | B |
| 45. | A |
| 46. | B |
| 47. | C |
| 48. | C |
| 49. | B |
| 50. | B |
| 51. | D |
| 52. | B |
| 53. | B |
| 54. | D |
| 55. | C |
| 56. | C |
| 57. | A |
| 58. | A |
| 59. | B |
| 60. | B |
| 61. | D |
| 62. | B |
| 63. | A |
| 64. | B |
| 65. | B |
| 66. | A |
| 67. | B |
| 68. | A |
| 69. | D |
| 70. | A |
| 71. | B |

**CHAPTER 14**

| | |
|---|---|
| 72. | C |

**CHAPTER 15**

| | |
|---|---|
| 1. | A |
| 2. | B |
| 3. | A |
| 4. | B |
| 5. | B |
| 6. | D |
| 7. | A |
| 8. | B |
| 9. | A |
| 10. | B |
| 11. | A |
| 12. | A |
| 13. | C |
| 14. | C |
| 15. | A |
| 16. | B |
| 17. | C |
| 18. | C |
| 19. | D |
| 20. | B |
| 21. | A |
| 22. | B |
| 23. | C |
| 24. | B |
| 25. | C |
| 26. | D |
| 27. | C |
| 28. | A |
| 29. | A |
| 30. | B |
| 31. | B |
| 32. | C |
| 33. | A |
| 34. | A |
| 35. | A |
| 36. | D |

**CHAPTER 16**

| | |
|---|---|
| 1. | A |
| 2. | D |
| 3. | C |
| 4. | A |
| 5. | A |
| 6. | C |
| 7. | C |
| 8. | B |

| | |
|---|---|
| 9. | C |
| 10. | C |
| 11. | C |
| 12. | B |
| 13. | A |
| 14. | B |
| 15. | C |
| 16. | C |
| 17. | C |
| 18. | D |
| 19. | A |
| 20. | B |
| 21. | D |
| 22. | C |
| 23. | C |
| 24. | A |
| 25. | C |
| 26. | C |
| 27. | A |
| 28. | B |
| 29. | B |
| 30. | A |
| 31. | B |
| 32. | B |
| 33. | D |
| 34. | B |
| 35. | C |
| 36. | D |
| 37. | C |
| 38. | B |
| 39. | A |
| 40. | A |
| 41. | A |
| 42. | A |
| 43. | C |
| 44. | B |
| 45. | B |
| 46. | D |
| 47. | B |
| 48. | C |
| 49. | B |
| 50. | D |
| 51. | A |
| 52. | G |
| 53. | C |
| 54. | E |
| 55. | B |
| 56. | D |
| 57. | F |

**CHAPTER 17**

| | |
|---|---|
| 1. | A |
| 2. | B |
| 3. | C |
| 4. | A |
| 5. | C |
| 6. | D |
| 7. | B |
| 8. | A |
| 9. | C |
| 10. | C |
| 11. | B |
| 12. | A |
| 13. | D |
| 14. | D |
| 15. | C |
| 16. | B |
| 17. | B |
| 18. | B |
| 19. | A |
| 20. | A |
| 21. | C |
| 22. | A |
| 23. | D |
| 24. | A |
| 25. | C |
| 26. | B |
| 27. | C |
| 28. | A |

**CHAPTER 18**

| | |
|---|---|
| 1. | D |
| 2. | B |
| 3. | B |
| 4. | B |
| 5. | C |
| 6. | A |
| 7. | B |
| 8. | A |
| 9. | C |
| 10. | D |
| 11. | B |
| 12. | D |
| 13. | B |
| 14. | C |
| 15. | B |
| 16. | C |
| 17. | C |
| 18. | D |
| 19. | A |
| 20. | D |
| 21. | A |

| | |
|---|---|
| 22. | A |
| 23. | D |
| 24. | A |
| 25. | C |
| 26. | C |
| 27. | D |
| 28. | C |
| 29. | A |
| 30. | C |
| 31. | B |
| 32. | B |
| 33. | A |
| 34. | D |

**CHAPTER 19**

| | |
|---|---|
| 1. | D |
| 2. | B |
| 3. | A |
| 4. | B |
| 5. | B |
| 6. | B |
| 7. | A |
| 8. | D |
| 9. | C |
| 10. | A |
| 11. | A |
| 12. | C |
| 13. | C |
| 14. | B |
| 15. | B |
| 16. | B |
| 17. | D |
| 18. | B |
| 19. | A |
| 20. | B |
| 21. | A |
| 22. | A |
| 23. | A |
| 24. | C |
| 25. | A |
| 26. | B |
| 27. | B |
| 28. | D |
| 29. | B |
| 30. | A |
| 31. | C |
| 32. | A |
| 33. | C |
| 34. | C |
| 35. | B |
| 36. | C |

## CHAPTER 19

| | |
|---|---|
| 37. | A |
| 38. | B |
| 39. | A |
| 40. | B |
| 41. | B |
| 42. | A |
| 43. | C |
| 44. | A |
| 45. | B |
| 46. | D |
| 47. | B |
| 48. | C |
| 49. | A |
| 50. | B |
| 51. | C |

## CHAPTER 20

| | |
|---|---|
| 1. | C |
| 2. | A |
| 3. | A |
| 4. | B |
| 5. | A |
| 6. | C |
| 7. | C |
| 8. | B |
| 9. | C |
| 10. | A |
| 11. | A |
| 12. | A |
| 13. | A |
| 14. | B |
| 15. | D |
| 16. | D |
| 17. | A |
| 18. | B |
| 19. | C |
| 20. | D |
| 21. | B |
| 22. | C |
| 23. | C |
| 24. | A |
| 25. | B |
| 26. | B |
| 27. | A |
| 28. | B |
| 29. | D |
| 30. | C |
| 31. | C |
| 32. | B |

| | |
|---|---|
| 33. | C |
| 34. | D |
| 35. | A |
| 36. | D |
| 37. | B |
| 38. | C |
| 39. | C |
| 40. | B |
| 41. | B |
| 42. | D |
| 43. | B |
| 44. | C |
| 45. | C |
| 46. | A |
| 47. | C |
| 48. | B |
| 49. | A |
| 50. | B |
| 51. | C |
| 52. | D |